TURNING OFF

ING OFF

BREAST CANCER

TURNING OFF

BREAST CANCER

A Personalized Approach to Nutrition
and Detoxification in Prevention and Healing

DANIELLA CHACE, MS, CN

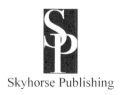

Skyhorse Publishing

Skyhorse Publishing books may be purchased in bulk at special discounts for sales promotion, corporate gifts, fund-raising, or educational purposes. Special editions can also be created to specifications. For details, contact the Special Sales Department, Skyhorse Publishing, 307 West 36th Street, 11th Floor, New York, NY 10018 or info@skyhorsepublishing.com.

Skyhorse® and Skyhorse Publishing® are registered trademarks of Skyhorse Publishing, Inc.®, a Delaware corporation.

Visit our website at www.skyhorsepublishing.com.

10 9 8 7 6 5 4 3 2 1

Library of Congress Cataloging-in-Publication Data is available on file.

Cover design by Georgia Morrissey
Cover photo courtesy of Shutterstock
Interior art by Julie Read, www.artbyjulieread.com

Print ISBN: 978-1-63220-445-5
Ebook ISBN: 978-1-63220-758-6

Printed in the United States of America

CONTENTS

Dedication and Acknowledgments   vii

Introduction   ix

Chapter One: How to Use this Book   1

Chapter Two: Genetics   3

Chapter Three: Detoxify   15

Chapter Four: Nutrition   43

Chapter Five: Microbial Health   89

Chapter Six: Supplements   99

Chapter Seven: Self-Care   111

References   119

Glossaries   147

Resources   160

About the Author   162

Index   163

Dedication

Linda Landkammer, my dear mother,
who inspires and guides by example.

Acknowledgments

Patrick Jennings, for his support during this intense period of research and writing.

Helen Gray, for her proofreading and endless enthusiasm for nutrition and healing.

Bonnie Story, Keven Elliff, and Tina Amen, who are the experts I rely on to make it all happen.

Abigail Gehring, my editor at Skyhorse, for her vision and commitment to this book.

Dr. David S. Moore, Dr. Neil Barnard, Dr. Colin Campbell, Dr. Joel Fuhrman, Dr. Barry Boyd, Dr. Barbara McClintock, Dr. David C. Seldin, Dr. Gail E. Sonenshein, Dr. Stefano Monti, Dr. Charlotte Kuperwasser, Dr. Andrea Girman, Dr. Bradford Weeks, Dr. Lise Alchuler, Dr. Walter Crinnion, Dr. Sandra Poling, and Dr. Paul Rubin, who blazed the trail to this new era of health care.

INTRODUCTION

TREATING THE CAUSE RATHER THAN THE SYMPTOMS

We find ourselves in a tremendously exciting time in integrative oncology care. There is a wealth of new breast cancer research from clinical trials around the world, providing many of the answers to our questions about the factors that trigger, promote, heal, and prevent breast cancer. We now have a much fuller picture of breast cancer and know that it is an issue of internal cellular miscommunication caused by toxins, nutrient deficiencies, and microbial imbalance.

A MULTIFACTORIAL DISEASE

As breast cancer is a complex condition in which many factors play a role, targeted interventions must be used to correct these varied imbalances to effectively reverse its trajectory. These interventions decrease risk and increase healing and prevention.

ENVIRONMENT AND LIFESTYLE

Only about 25 percent of breast cancer cases result from inherited genes that carry a risk for cancer. Most cases of breast cancer result from changes caused by environmental and lifestyle factors. An imbalance in one area—such as lack of sleep, exercise, nutrients, gut flora, and social connection or an excess of toxins, hormones, stress, or medications—can increase the risk of breast cancer, and a combination of two or more imbalances substantially increases risk.

GENETIC TRIGGERS

There was a long-held belief that genes had a permanent plan for our biology. It is now understood that many of our genetic markers for cancer will not necessarily be "expressed" and that environmental factors such as toxins, nutrients, and hormones control whether our genes will direct our cells to develop cancer.

POLYMORPHISMS

Poly (many) morphisms (distortions) are abnormal codes in our genes that are affected by unhealthy chemicals such as toxins and healthy chemicals such as nutrients. We have all been exposed to toxins through our environment and nutrients through our food so our genes are in various phases of distortions. Toxins create weaknesses in our genes that have the potential to turn on breast cancer pathways, which means they can trigger gene expression. Once a gene has been triggered it then expresses directives such as cell growth. The affects that these triggers have on genes is the science of epigenetics.

Epigenetic tests can identify potential problems in our personal genetic code. This gives us the opportunity to address these specific weaknesses directly. Supporting our bodies in overcoming these inefficiencies can play a significant role in reducing cancer development.

BREAST CANCER EPIGENETICS

Specific nutrients and toxins can turn cancer cells off or on. For example, piperine, found in concentrated amounts in black pepper, has an epigenetic effect, which can change the expression of genes, even ones that are programmed for cancer. And peppercorns are just one of hundreds of foods that have been found to contain nutrients that target breast cancer.

Over the last decade there has been a tremendous surge in research identifying the nutrients that directly change the course of breast cancer. A few examples of nutrients that play key roles include folate, vitamin D, carotenoids, melatonin, selenium, flavonols, and sulfur compounds.

Many of the foods found to affect breast cancer provide their benefits via normalization of DNA methylation, which is the key that turns genes off and on. Microbes are the living organisms that exist in the trillions throughout our digestive systems. They live symbiotically with us, in our gut and on our bodies. These organisms are necessary for our health and we need them to flourish to support the methylation process and to help us absorb food nutrients.

THE MICROBIOME

New microbiome research has increased our understanding of the role of microbes in disease and has shown us that our bodies are living laboratories of symbiotic and pathogenic bacteria. These organisms play key roles in cancer development, cognitive function, nutrient metabolism, protection from infectious agents, and immune regulation.

BREAST CARCINOGENS

There are a handful of common toxins that are known carcinogens that target breast cells. These include heavy metals, phthalates, and polyaromatic hydrocarbons. Because these toxins are so prevalent in our modern lives, and breast cancer is such a common health problem, we should all be taking measures to avoid exposure to toxins. Those with breast cancer are often found to have significantly higher levels of one or more of these compounds in their bodies.

While this indicates that we need changes in environmental regulation to protect us all from these carcinogens, it more directly confirms that testing for toxins should be a primary strategy in all breast cancer healing plans.

PERSONALIZED APPROACH

Applying nutrition, toxicology, epigenetics, and microbiology in breast cancer care is an effective strategy because imbalances in these areas create the environment that allows breast cancer cell development.

EVIDENCE-INFORMED DECISIONS

The recent research that has brought us to an understanding of these known causes of breast cancer is absolutely thrilling. As a practitioner, I find these discoveries, and the protocols based on them, to be empowering for patients, who now have the ability to remediate many of these issues in their own bodies. This book describes this exciting new research and breaks it down into concrete steps that can be taken to reduce risk and heal breast cancer.

TURNING OFF

ING OFF

BREAST CANCER

Chapter One

HOW TO USE THIS BOOK

Use this as your personal workbook. You may choose to simply glance at each section, read the chapter summary, and dive right into the action steps. The checklists at the end of each chapter are reminders of the steps to take based on the recommendations in each chapter. They include actions, such as replacing toxic products in your home with non-toxic alternatives, ordering lab test kits, and shopping for specific nutrient-dense foods. This way you can get started immediately. Later, when you want to learn more, you can take the time to read through the science behind the recommendations.

Alternatively, if you want to start by reading about the science, you may want keep a pen handy so you can underline the areas that apply to you, make notes in the margins, and circle the sections you want to refer back to later. For example, if you have an estrogen-receptor-positive subtype, you may circle the recommendations that apply to ER+ as you come across them. Also, while reading about supplements, you may want to check to see if you're taking enough CoQ10, for example. You could then circle the recommended daily dose to remind yourself to compare it to your current intake. You may also want to highlight foods in the sections that sound appealing to you or just make a copy of the grocery list provided. Check off the foods you would like to start eating more of and take it with you to the grocery store.

You will encounter many scientific and medical terms throughout the book. You can use the Glossaries section in the back as a reference to look up terms as you run into them. The studies and research used to inform the recommendations throughout this book are provided in the References section.

Chapter Two

GENETICS

Genetics play a role in breast cancer development. Details about your personal genetic background, family history, and susceptibility to environmental factors can be revealed with laboratory tests. They identify risk factors and subtypes, such as cellular sensitivity to estrogen. These distinct molecular subtypes differ in their responsiveness to therapeutic and preventive agents, so diagnosis is critical.

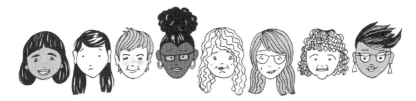

GENETIC TESTS

These tests help practitioners create more targeted and personalized treatment. Genetic tests give us the ability to meet the needs of an individual's physiology and genetic makeup. They provide personalized details about how medications, environmental toxins, and nutrients will affect your breast cancer. These tests also determine the degree of risk from exposure to environmental toxins. Using this information, your risk level can be mitigated through diet, detoxification, nutrient therapy, and microbial supplementation.

One of the primary differences in subtypes is in their responsiveness to hormones. Knowing what type you have helps you evaluate the importance of avoiding hormone exposure from estrogenic foods, medications, and toxins that pose a greater risk for those with hormone-sensitive cancers.

In contrast, some breast cancer subtypes, such as estrogen receptor negative (ER-), do not respond to hormones but do respond to other compounds, such as nutrients and toxins, which are powerful controllers in these specific subtypes.

ENDOCRINE-DISRUPTING CHEMICALS (EDCs)

When compounds interfere with our hormones, they are affecting our endocrine systems. Many endocrine-disrupting chemicals (EDCs) are ubiquitous in the environment today, which means that exposure is likely. Some of these occur naturally, while others are man-made.

Many of these EDCs have estrogenic properties, which means that they mimic the action of estrogen in our bodies. Ongoing exposure to EDCs has been found to increase the development of specific endocrine-related diseases, including breast cancer.

Compounds such as phthalates, parabens, and heavy metals are known as *xenoestrogens, xeno-* meaning foreign to our bodies. They have the ability to communicate and signal our cells and our genes in the same way as our own natural hormones (Knower et al., 2013). When we ingest, inhale, or absorb them, our cells recognize them as hormones.

BREAST CANCER SUBTYPES

This first step in understanding the internal imbalances that lead to your breast cancer is genetic testing. Genetic tests help determine risk factors and subtypes. Some forms of breast cancer, or subtypes, are hormone receptor positive, such as HER2+, AR+, ER+, and PR+, while some forms of breast cancer are hormone receptor negative, for example ER-, PR-, and AR-.

BREAST CANCER SUBTYPES AND SPECIFIC DIETARY NEEDS

Hormone driven breast cancer (also known as hormone-mediated, hormone-sensitive, or hormone-dependent breast cancer) refers to any cancer that is triggered or made worse by the action of hormones such as estrogen, progesterone, or androgen. These types of cancer respond well to epigenetic therapies (Basse et al., 2014).

ESTROGEN RECEPTOR POSITIVE

More than two-thirds of breast cancers express the estrogen receptor (ER+) and depend on estrogen for growth and survival. Historically, therapies targeting ER+ either inhibit estrogen or block its production and play a central role in the treatment of ER+ breast cancers of all stages (Balleine et al., 2012). Newer, more specific approaches also include avoiding estrogenic toxins and foods.

Dietary therapy that targets the specific needs of these subtypes is one of the most effective strategies we have in personalized medicine. For example, saturated fats increase the risk for ER+ cancer development and growth (Sieri et al., 2014). Therefore, those with a family history and/or with a diagnosis of ER+ should avoid eating saturated fats.

Food nutrients have been found to be especially effective for certain subtypes. Carnosic acid from rosemary, for example, inhibits the growth of ER- breast cancer cells (Einbond et al., 2012). Carnosic acid has the ability to activate the expression of several different genes involved in breast cancer protection, and also enhances the biosynthesis of glutathione, a nutrient that helps us excrete toxins known to stimulate breast cancer development. It also triggers apoptosis, the programmed cell death of breast cancer cells.

The combination of certain food nutrients makes them even more effective, as is the case with carnosic acid and curcumin. Curcumin is the bioactive compound in turmeric. Curcumin directly affects enzymes involved in epigenetic mechanisms that inhibit breast cancer.

Carnosic acid (from rosemary) has been shown to be more effective in preventing and treating breast cancer when combined with curcumin (from turmeric).

TRIPLE NEGATIVE BREAST CANCER (TNBC)

Triple-negative breast cancer (TNBC) refers to any breast cancer that does express the genes for estrogen receptor (ER), progesterone receptor (PR) or Her2/neu. It comprises approximately 15 percent of breast cancers and is particularly aggressive and hard to treat. Many patients with TNBC relapse quickly and commonly develop metastases. As the name suggests, TNBCs are not hormone modified. They have a higher rate of relapse in the first five years but lower relapse rates after five years compared to hormone-modified breast cancers.

The current oncology treatments available for TNBC are highly toxic. There are significant advantages to applying all of the effective dietary and detoxification strategies known to date for this subtype.

New studies of TNBC and food nutrients have illuminated the powerful effects of specific whole foods in the healing of TNBC. For example, blueberries contain pterostilbene, an anticancer agent that acts on TNBC. A lab study found that mice fed a 5 percent whole blueberry powder diet had significantly smaller tumors, less ulceration, and significantly fewer metastases to the lymph nodes than mice fed their normal diet.

It has also been recently discovered that naringenin, which is a major flavonoid found in citrus fruit, concentrates in breast tissue, inhibits cell proliferation, and promotes apoptosis. This nutrient is now considered an important addition in integrative care for treatment of TNBC. Naringenin also provides protective effects against damage from compounds in plastics, such as BPA.

Omega-3 fatty acids have been found to affect TNBC via multiple cellular mechanisms leading to inhibition of proliferation and induction of apoptosis. A specific omega-3 fatty acid called docosahexaenoic acid (DHA) was tested on human TNBC and was found to significantly inhibit cell proliferation (20–90 percent reduction). This inhibitory effect was more pronounced on TNBC than any other type of cancer (Pogash et al., 2015).

Green tea is another food that contains powerful nutrients that support healing of TNBC. Daily intake of green tea boosts EGCG, which directly affects epigenetic pathways and improves biomarkers involved in hormone-receptor-negative breast cancers.

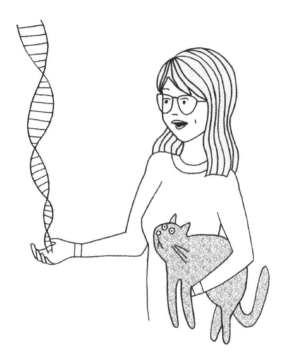

EPIGENETICS

Many of the anticancer actions of food nutrients take place through epigenetics, which is an important mechanism by which external factors affect genetic expression. The term epigenetics, which comes from *epi-* (meaning *above*) and *genetics* (the study of DNA coding), is a fairly new field of research based on the discovery that the individual genetic map is malleable. External and internal environmental factors (present in the body as molecules) can turn the expression of gene coding off or on.

Toxins, nutrients, hormones, and microbes play a major role in the development of cancer. We have also learned which molecules, such as nutrients and bacteria, turn off the cancer cascade in various ways.

EPIGENETIC TOXINS

Toxins can act as genetic triggers, causing unhealthy epigenetic effects. Breast cancer genes may be turned on by exposure to chemical toxins, such as those in smoke, pesticides, plastics, and processed foods. For example, many heavy metals, such as aluminum, mercury, and lead, have the ability to increase estrogen-related gene expression in human breast cancer cells. Parabens and phthalates also have the ability to directly affect breast cancer genes and can stimulate the growth and spread of breast cancer cells (Singh et al., 2012; Park et al., 2012).

EPIGENETIC NUTRIENTS

Whole foods and supplements provide nutrients that have a positive effect on DNA methylation. Methyl molecules turn genes on and off. Methyl donor nutrients include folate, vitamin B12, methionine, choline, and betaine. Thus, epigenetics can be thought of as the management of genetic activity. These actions involve molecular messages that affect cancer in various ways including enzymatic reactions, suppression of tumor growth, cellular division, genetic repair, and apoptosis (programmed cancer cell destruction).

Although DNA remains unaltered, epigenetic changes effect gene expression. Genes in our DNA hold the code for certain actions but can remain dormant or inactive until turned on. Various stimulants, such as bioactive food components, contain the trigger.

These nutrients contain molecules that have the ability to fit into receptor sites on genes that either hinder or trigger the expression of these genes. The molecular component that fits into the receptor sites is called a methyl group.

Many of the nutrients that influence genes do this by way of methyl groups that have an epigenetic effect by turning off genetic pathways that lead to cancer.

POLYMORPHISMS AND BREAST CANCER

About 5–10 percent of breast cancer cases are due to genes inherited from one's parents. But most of the genes that pose a risk for breast cancer have been triggered by chemical reactions leading to polymorphic changes.

Polymorphism, meaning *many mutations,* are the DNA variations. These variations are also known as SNPs, which is pronounced "snips" (single nucleotide polymorphisms). SNPs often identify a weakened resistance to disease. They are diagnosed through genetic testing. SNP tests help us identify areas of risk, detect problems early, and classify diseases. They can also guide the use of targeted therapy.

Therefore, identifying these SNPs and implementing therapy to compensate for them is a primary healing strategy. For example, those with BReast CAncer (BRCA) have mutations in either the BRCA1 or BRCA2 genes that produce tumor suppressor proteins. The diagnoses of BRCA1 or BRCA2 substantially increase the likelihood that additional genetic alterations that can lead to cancer will occur. Epigenetic testing and remediations are particularly important for this risk group.

Testing for these biomarkers offers a roadmap to strengthen areas of risk. SNP tests identify weaknesses in an individual's genetic makeup and provide a roadmap to address them directly. For example, when

SNPs are identified, we can reduce the damage they might cause by increasing specific nutrients and detoxifying certain compounds from the body.

A DetoxiGenomic Profile is a SNP test done with a sample of your genetic material. The test is performed with just a few cells taken from the inside of the cheek with a cotton swab. This profile tests for a variety of SNPs involved in the clearance of environmental toxins that affect breast cancer development, such as COMT, GSTM, and GSTP.

A reduction in the COMT (catechol-O-methyltransferase) enzyme increases the risk for impaired ability to break down estrogen and stress hormones, such as cortisol. For those with hormone-sensitive breast cancer, this is significant, as estrogen may not be efficiently eliminated from the body.

If you have this SNP, you can reduce its effects by minimizing sustained mental and environmental stress. You can also make sure that you are taking in the nutrients needed to support this enzyme pathway, which include B vitamins, magnesium, and protein.

If your test results show that you have a weakness in COMT, a saliva hormone panel that includes sex hormones and cortisol will help you and your healthcare team understand the underlying factors in your cancer development. With these details you will then know whether your hormone levels need to be monitored.

Glutathione S-transferases (GSTs) are other liver enzymes responsible for detoxifying certain breast carcinogens, such as solvents, herbicides, pesticides, polycyclic aromatic hydrocarbons (PAHs), steroids (hormones), and heavy metals (metalloestrogens). This genetic mutation holds an ever greater risk for those with hormone-sensitive cancers because it reduces the ability to break down hormones and hormone imitators, such as heavy metals.

Once you know that you have this mutation, you can directly address the issues it causes. For example, supplements, such as methionine, N-acetyl cysteine, glutamine, glycine, magnesium, and vitamin B6, support the clearance of certain breast cell toxins. Also you can reduce excess hormones by eating brassica vegetables daily.

A GSTP polymorphism indicates a reduced production of the important detoxification nutrient glutathione and the detox enzymes that need glutathione. This SNP is associated with an increased risk for breast cancer that is compounded by exposure to PAHs, such as smoke and certain chemicals and metals. To compensate for this mutation you can minimize exposure to cigarette smoke, charred food, herbicides, fungicides, insect sprays, industrial solvents, and heavy metals.

You can also make dietary changes to support this SNP. Brassica vegetables contain the biochemical isothiocyanate, which have a supportive effect on the GSTP genetic polymorphism. Increasing dietary consumption of the brassica vegetables such as broccoli, cauliflower, cabbage, kale, and Brussels sprouts, as well as allium vegetables such as onions, leeks, and garlic can all increase glutathione activity and offset the risk caused by this mutation. And consuming antioxidant foods such as wild blueberries, herbs, turmeric, and citrus fruits can reduce the oxidative stress inherently caused by this SNP. Many nutrients that support production of glutathione can be taken as supplements, which include alpha lipoic acid, milk thistle, and taurine.

EPIGENETIC MICROBES

Fungi and bacteria play a more complex role in epigenetics. Bacteria break down estrogen, reducing the amount of estrogen metabolites circulating in the body, which in turn reduces the amount of estrogen triggering receptor sites. Microbes also do this by breaking down the estrogen via enterohepatic circulation as well as metabolizing phytoestrogens that either come from the foods we eat or from the hormones that we produce internally.

Microbes also play a key role in methylation. They are able to liberate methyl groups from foods and nutrients, which makes these methyl groups available to methylate genes, thus turning them down or off. This is a very important step in reducing the potential risk from genes that trigger breast cancer.

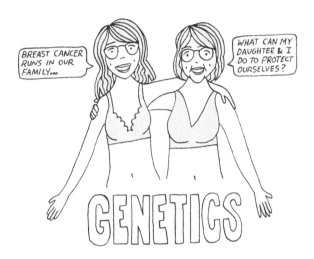

■ STRATEGY: GENETICS CHAPTER

Your oncologist will run tests to determine your tumor markers and subtype. If your cancer cells are sensitive to hormones, you can reduce your exposure to hormones in various ways such as discontinuing hormone replacement therapy, avoiding plant estrogens, and avoiding hormone-mimicking chemicals.

CHECKLIST
- Ask your oncologist if you have a hormone-sensitive type of breast cancer.
- Contact a physician (MD or ND) who can order the genomic profiles that identity polymorphisms (SNPs). For example, estrogen metabolism tests including CYP, GST, GSTP, GSTM and COMT.
- If you have a hormone-sensitive subtype, consider having the EstroGenomic Profile (Genova Diagnostics), which evalu-

ates the genes that modulate estrogen metabolism, including CYP, GST, and COMT. These estrogen metabolism SNPs focus on the Phase 1 enzymes involved in the formation of anticarcinogenic metabolites, such as hydroxyestrone.

- Ask your doctor to test your level of methylation nutrients, which include vitamin panels, amino acids, choline, and betaine. One such test is the ION (Individual Optimal Nutrition) Profile (Genova Diagnostics) which includes all of these as well as fatty acids.

For more support in locating a physician, finding these tests, and keeping informed about nutrients that help specific subtypes, visit www.daniellachace.com.

Chapter Three

DETOXIFY

We know that most cases of breast cancer have no inherited component, which means there are other reasons that it develops. Finding those reasons has been a focus for integrative and environmental medical professionals over the last few decades, and they have done a tremendous job of identifying the toxins and imbalances that contribute to the development of breast cancer.

We not only know which toxins are carcinogenic but also which common toxins have the ability to trigger the development of breast cancer. Toxins are compounds that have negative health effects. These include natural elements, chemicals, smoke, and gases. We are exposed to them through our air, food, water, homes, and environment.

To "detox" means to actively remove toxins from the body. Generally, a detox is a practice of consciously removing common toxins from our homes and diet. These often include cigarettes, alcohol, red meat, sugar, dairy, and gluten.

Toxins that enter our bodies, either through our lungs, skin, or digestive tracts, enter our blood stream, where they then flow throughout our bodies. As they pass through the liver, enzymes are secreted that break them down so that they can be eliminated through our stool, urine, and sweat.

Environmental medicine researchers have identified breast cancer toxins and effective detoxification for each. There are three ways to address these. First, request the lab tests that look for these compounds in your body. Second, assume you have had exposure due to the ubiquity of toxins, and learn how to avoid future exposure. Third, learn what foods and nutrients are necessary to clean these toxins from your body.

LAB TESTS FOR BREAST CANCER TOXINS

In my clinical practice, I always recommend that those with breast cancer, or even those with a genetic risk for developing breast cancer, have the tests. I can then directly address the specific toxicities rather than having to consider the potential exposure for all of the breast toxins. Lab tests ultimately allow us to save time and money as they provide details about the specific compounds and the concentration of contamination in each individual.

Within the general population, some of us have more exposure to certain compounds than others. Also, we may be exposed to numerous chemicals, which has a cumulative effect. When we think of toxins, we might conjure images of smoke stacks, gasoline, waste sites, and bottles of chemicals displaying a skull and crossbones. But toxicologists have discovered that we actually have a much higher exposure to dangerous toxins inside our homes than we do outside our homes.

Individual toxicity levels radically effect disease outcomes, therefore an awareness of known breast cancer carcinogens provide an opportunity for detoxification and reduction in exposure. The evidence that has emerged from studies of environmental factors involved in breast cancer point to new areas of research. First, breast cancer is now recognized as a developmental disease, with greater susceptibility across the lifetime, beginning in the womb, during puberty and the early reproductive years, and up to diagnosis.

Research has identified common chemicals that activate biological pathways involved in breast cancer development, such as genotoxic chemicals that cause mammary gland tumors and those that act as hormone disruptors that interact with the estrogen receptor and promote tumor proliferation.

Learning about toxins that are all around us may feel alarming, but learning which toxins pose the greatest risk for your specific genetic makeup gives you the power to take steps to avoid exposure and reduce these compounds in your body.

BROMINE

Bromine is a widespread toxin that is a potential antagonist in the development of breast cancer. Bromine has been linked to cancer, obesity, and diabetes development (Andra et al., 2014).

The use of brominated flame retardants and incineration of bromine-containing materials has led to an increase in polybrominated compounds in the environment. It is so widely used commercially that our environment is laced with bromine and bromine compounds. Random sampling found that these compounds are affecting humans and wildlife. They have been detected in human blood, adipose tissue, and breast milk.

Bromine is a toxin and interferes with our immune function. Immune suppression is a side effect of bromine exposure (Frawley et al., 2014). Also bromine impairs mitochondrial function, thus impairing energy production in the body (Pazin et al., 2015).

Bromine compounds are suspected of creating iodine deficiency, which is associated with the development of breast cancer. When we are exposed to bromine, it has the ability to bond to iodine receptors, preventing iodine from being absorbed and thus causing the potential for iodine deficiency. Iodine deficiency is linked to breast cancer development as iodine is necessary for healthy cell development and secretory cells of the breasts. Also iodine deficiency allows heavy metals to bind in breast tissue, which increases the risk for the development of breast cancer.

Sources

Bromine is an industrial chemical used in large volumes in fire retardants and baked goods. Bromine compounds have long technical names that reflect their chemical composition and are better known by their acronyms, for example:

Brominated flame retardants (BFRs)

Polybrominated diphenyl ethers (PBDEs)

Tetrabromobisphenol A (TBBPA)

Hexabromocyclododecane (HBCD)

Polybrominated biphenyls (PBBs)

PBDE (bromide) interfere with biochemical processes and accumulate in body tissues. Fire retardants are commonly used in mattresses, carpeting, furniture, car interiors, and hair dyes.

Potassium bromate is used as an additive in most commercial bread and baked goods. Read bread labels and look for terms that indicate bromine use, which include bromated flour, enriched flour, or dough conditioners.

Environmental medicine practitioners suspect that many people are experiencing bromine toxicity symptoms, which include skin rashes, severe acne, loss of appetite, abdominal pain, fatigue, metallic taste, and cardiac arrhythmias. Reduce exposure to bromine by avoiding commercial baked goods, opting instead for organic, whole-grain baked goods.

If you spend considerable time around other potential sources of exposure, such as your car interior, carpet at home or work, or have a non-natural mattress, try to increase ventilation as much as possible. Wiping down the windows and interior of your car will help remove some of the bromine dust that accumulates as a film.

Avoiding bromine from carpeting requires either daily ventilation or removal of the carpet. Use an organic mattress pad or purchase an all-natural rubber mattress. We spend many hours a day with our faces close to the mattress, so it can be a considerable source of bromine.

NUTRIENT PROTECTION

Potassium bromate is the form of bromine added to commercial baked goods as a dough conditioner. Antioxidant nutrients, such as phenols and flavonoids as well as minerals such as potassium, calcium, magnesium, and zinc have been found to protect against the toxic effects of potassium bromate (Saad et al., 2014).

Bromine Sources

- Flame Retardants: Bromine compounds used in fabrics, carpets, upholstery, and mattresses.
- Pesticides: Specifically methyl bromide, used mainly on strawberries.
- Plastics: Bromide plastics are used to make computers.
- Dough Conditioners: Bakery goods and some flours contain a dough conditioner called potassium bromate.
- Soft Drinks: Citrus-flavored sodas, including Mountain Dew, Gatorade, Sun Drop, Squirt, and Fresca, contain bromine in the form of brominated vegetable oils (BVOs).
- Medications: Asthma inhalers such as Atrovent Inhaler, Atrovent Nasal Spray, Pro-Banthine (for ulcers), and some anesthesia agents contain bromine.
- Pool Sanitizers: Bromine-based hot tub and swimming pool treatments are used in place of chlorine to kill bacteria and contaminants.
- Personal Care Products: Toothpastes, mouthwash, and gargles contain potassium bromate as an antiseptic and astringent. Sodium bromate is found in permanent wave neutralizers and hair dye formulas.
- Vegetable Oils: Bromine is found in brominated vegetable oil.

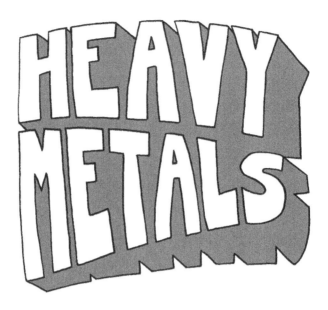

Heavy Metals and Breast Cancer

Heavy metals include aluminum, antimony, arsenic, barium, bismuth, cadmium, cesium, chromium, gadolinium, gallium, lead, mercury, nickel, niobium, platinum, rubidium, thallium, tin, tungsten, and uranium.

Metals are natural elements that can be highly toxic in certain forms and especially harmful for those who have been exposed to concentrated amounts over a period of time. Heavy metals, which include mercury and lead, can block mineral absorption, cause neurological problems, and be particularly toxic to those with estrogen-sensitive breast cancer. Metals are some of the most common toxins in our environment and of particular concern for those who don't have the genetic ability to excrete them efficiently.

Heavy metals have been suspected as a primary risk factor in breast cancer development. Recent research in which concentrations of heavy metals have been found in different parts of breast cancer tissues substantiate this theory (Mohammadi et al., 2014). They have been found to pose an even higher risk for those with estrogen-sensitive cancers as they can stimulate the growth of estrogen-sensitive cells and tumors (Bryne et al., 2013).

Sources

Our environment contains heavy metals, so our risk of exposure and contamination is high. Heavy metals are found naturally in the earth and become concentrated as a result of human activities. Metals are often found in concentration at mining sites, in industrial wastes, vehicle emissions, lead batteries, agricultural fertilizers, and treated wood. But they are also present in our food, such as mercury in fish, in our food packaging, such as aluminum soda cans, and even in our dental fillings.

Metalloestrogens

These metals have the potential to add to the estrogenic burden of the human breast by mimicking estrogen in the absence of estradiol, which activates estrogen receptors (Darbre, 2006).

Metalloestrogens that have been identified so far include aluminum, antimony, arsenite, barium, cadmium, a specific form of chromium, cobalt, copper, lead, mercury, nickel, selenite, tin, and vanadate (a form of vanadium).

Estrogenicity

There is a range of estrogenicity in these metals, which is to say that some have a stronger estrogenic effect than others on cells.

Accumulation in the Body

Heavy metals become toxic when they are not metabolized by the body and accumulate in the soft tissues, kidneys, and liver. Heavy metals may enter the body through food, water, air, or absorption through the skin in agricultural, manufacturing, pharmaceutical, industrial, or residential settings. Amalgam fillings in our teeth contain mercury.

We are exposed to each metal in specific ways and can protect ourselves by avoiding the sources. Cadmium, nickel, and aluminum are often elevated in the urine of women with breast cancer at the time of diagnosis (Romanowicz-Makowska et al., 2011). This substantiates concerns in the environmental medical community that these metals play a role in the development of breast cancer.

The data suggest that both acute exposure to as well as gradual accumulation of heavy metals in the breast tissue may increase breast cancer growth. Environmental medicine experts are now recommending that breast cancer patients have an accurate evaluation of metal exposure. This can be determined with proper lab testing through urine or hair analysis tests, and subsequent chelation treatment may be employed to prevent and treat metal-related breast cancer.

Chelation treatment simply involves taking dietary supplements and foods that contain sulfur compounds that bind with the metals. This makes them easier to excrete through urine, stool, and sweat.

The stored metals recirculate in our blood, causing harm repeatedly. Our bodies are in a constant state of change and cell ™. Therefore, even though we can retain metals in our bodies for years, they tend to be released and restored repeatedly. For example, metals stored in our fat will become mobilized when we lose fat weight, and if our internal conditions are right, we might excrete some of these. Most of the population have well-functioning enzyme and methylation systems that are responsible for the excretion of metals through our urinary and digestive tracts. To a lesser degree, we store certain metals in our bone matrix. Bones degenerate and rebuild, releasing metals back into the blood, where they will be either shunted back into storage or excreted.

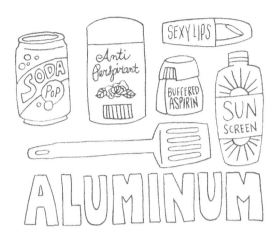

Aluminum

Aluminum becomes a toxin when it accumulates in tissues, disturbing natural physiologic processes. Those with a genetic weakness for clearance of heavy metals are at a higher risk for accumulation. There is emerging evidence suggesting aluminum accumulation in breast microenvironment is a possible risk factor for inflammatory breast cancer (IBC). Aluminum also acts as a metalloestrogen and can interfere with the function of estrogen receptors (Darbre et al., 2011). Aluminum has been found to cause oxidative stress and inflammation which both boost risk for breast cancer (Mannello et al., 2013).

Epigenetic Trigger
Aluminum exposure can affect our genetics as it also increases estrogen-related gene expression in human breast cancer cells.

Aluminum Forms
Aluminum chlorohydrate can be found in antiperspirants, lipsticks, and sunscreens. Aluminum in antiperspirants are concerning as aluminum can be absorbed through the skin, especially skin abraded

from shaving, and can migrate through the lymphatic system and accumulate in breast tissue. The increased risk for breast cancer from exposure to aluminum via antiperspirants has lead researchers to recommend that its use be reduced (Pineau et al., 2014).

Sodium aluminum phosphate and sodium aluminum sulfate are added as stabilizers to many processed foods including cake mixes and coffee creamers.

Aluminum Sources

Household sources of aluminum include aluminum cans, aluminum cooking utensils, baking soda, and food additives like dough conditioners, as well as food and drink packaging. Replace your aluminum kitchenwear with non-toxic alternatives, such as stainless steel, glass, or silicone.

Some of the most common personal care products that contain aluminum include antacids, buffered aspirin, some toothpastes, antiperspirants, medicines, lipsticks, and sunscreens.

Personal Care Alternatives

Natural herbal antiperspirants that act as antimicrobials are effective alternatives to aluminum-based products. Tea tree oil and grapefruit seed extract are effective natural antimicrobials used in alternative deodorant products. Look for deodorants that are free of aluminum, parabens, and phthalates.

Antimony

High antimony levels are associated with an increased risk of breast cancer. There is preliminary evidence that antimony plays a role in

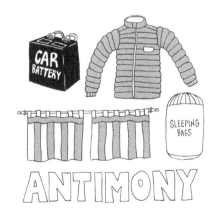

the etiology of BRCA1-associated breast cancer (Kotsopoulos et al., 2012).

Antimony Sources

Antimony is used in lead-acid batteries, solders, bullets, sheet and pipe metal, and bearings, and is a prominent additive in chlorine and bromine-containing fire retardants used commercially and in many household products. Antimony oxide is a form of antimony used in fire retardants. Textiles, paper, rubbers, upholstery, carpets, sleeping bags, automobile headers, and fabrics are treated with this type of fire retardant. Antimony trisulphide, another form of antimony, is used in the production of explosives, pigments, antimony salts, and ruby-colored glass.

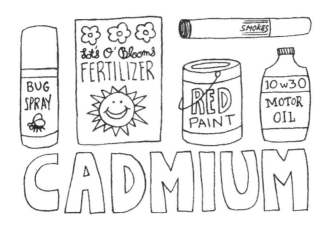

Cadmium

Cadmium is an environmental pollutant with well-studied estrogenic properties that has been linked to breast cancer development (Imran et al., 2014). Even low levels of cadmium exposure are associated with an increase in testosterone and a decrease in estradiol in postmenopausal women.

Researchers at the Gifu Medical School in Japan conducted a clever study to assess the correlation of cadmium in women who are diagnosed with breast cancer. They collected urine samples from 431 women who attended a breast cancer mass screening at their hospital. They used urine samples collected from the women after surgery, but before any cancer therapy. They compared these with the urine tests taken from those obtained at their normal screening visits. They found significantly higher cadmium levels in the women who had breast cancer. Their data suggests that exposure to cadmium is associated with a risk of breast cancer in Japanese women (Nagata et al., 2013).

Cadmium Sources

Cadmium is used in batteries, polyvinyl chloride plastics, and paint pigments. It can be found in soils because insecticides, fungicides, and commercial fertilizers that contain cadmium are used in agriculture. Cigarettes are a major source of exposure as cigarette paper is coated in cadmium to slow down the burning process. Lesser-known sources of exposure are dental alloys, electroplating, motor oil, and exhaust fumes.

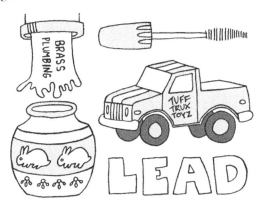

Lead

Lead is of particular concern as it has been shown to promote the development of existing breast tumors and it is the most prevalent heavy metal contaminant in the environment.

Lead Sources

Brass plumbing fixtures and copper soldered with lead can release particles into tap water. Glazes found on ceramics, china, and porcelain can contain lead. Products such as black eyeliner, mascara, lead-based paints, and children's painted toys may contain lead.

Risk Groups

Those with a depressed immune system from selenium deficiency who are exposed to lead have an increased cancer susceptibility.

Newly diagnosed IDC (infiltrating ductal carcinoma) patients in Nigeria were found to have higher levels of lead in their bodies compared to those from the same area who were found to be cancer-free.

It is also interesting to note that the Nigerian patients were found to have lead levels that correlated with the size of their tumors (Alatise et al., 2010). Conversely, it was discovered that the selenium levels in hair and blood were inversely correlated with the tumor volumes. Selenium and other minerals compete for the same binding sites as heavy metals and reduce the amount of metals that accumulate in the body. Selenium has also been found to have an antiproliferative effect on breast cancer cells.

Mercury

Symptoms of mercury toxicity include disturbed sensation and a lack of coordination, peripheral neuropathy, itching and burning skin, and pink cheeks, fingertips, and toes. Mercury is very toxic as it inhibits selenium-dependent enzymes.

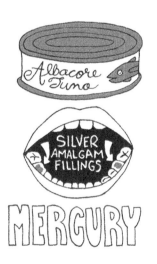

Symptoms of mercury poisoning include visual, hearing, and speech impairment and shedding or peeling skin. A person suffering from mercury poisoning may experience profuse sweating, tachycardia (persistently faster-than-normal heart beat), increased salivation, and hypertension (high blood pressure).

Mercury Sources

Sources of mercury toxicity include contaminated seafood, environmental pollution, and silver amalgam fillings. Seafood can contain heavy metals because they bio-accumulate in large, longer-living fish. Large fish are shark, swordfish, yellow fin, albacore tuna, and mackerel.

Other environmental exposures include vapors from the improper disposal of mercury-containing objects, for example, mercury thermometers and fluorescent lamps.

The World Health Organization has reported that the single largest contributor of mercury exposure to humans is amalgam fillings. Amalgam "silver" fillings are still being used in many dentistry practices to fill cavities caused by tooth decay. Amalgam fillings are made from a mixture of metals with approximately 50 percent mercury and the rest of the materials contain silver, tin, and copper. Amalgam fillings are a source of exposure because they release mercury vapors into our mouths. When we ingest small particles of metals from our fillings, we pass them through our digestive system without much absorption. But when we inhale the vapors from metals, they are absorbed through our lungs and into our blood where they can act as powerful toxins. Amalgam fillings release vapors at varying rates and increase when they come in contact with hot foods and liquids.

As we have learned about the health risks of amalgam fillings, more of us are considering having our amalgams removed. But removal of these fillings requires drilling, which creates the heat and friction that releases vapors. So this must be done by properly trained dental professionals known as biodynamic or biological dentists.

Patients making the decision whether or not to replace their amalgam fillings should be well informed about the potential risks versus benefits. Often the decision comes from a physician (MD or ND) who has determined that mercury exposure is detrimental to the patient's health.

Biological dentistry practices have special equipment and procedures that take these risks into consideration. Also dentists who specialize in amalgam removal take precautions, using a dental dam to protect the permeable lining of the cheeks and powerful ventilation systems to protect you from the inevitable vapors caused by the drilling needed for removal. There are safe removal protocols that have been developed by the International Academy of Oral Medicine and Toxicology (IAOMT).

To reduce the toxicity of the exposure to the metals, biological dentists also frequently use preliminary nutrients as a protective practice to help the body clear the metals. These nutrients may include vitamin C and N-acetyl cysteine.

Biological dentists replace the amalgams with gold, ceramic, or other alternate filling materials. Composite materials are also commonly used. The choice of material should be made carefully in each patient's situation.

Consult a biological dentist if you are concerned about the risk of exposure to mercury from your dental fillings and want to explore the option of removal.

Lab Tests for Heavy Metals

While blood tests will show acute exposure to metals and hair tests will reveal recent exposure, the most accurate lab test for 9 heavy metals in the body is a urine test, which provides more information about the total body load of these toxins. The test kit can be ordered through your health practitioner and the urine collection done at home. The test is called the Toxic

Element Clearance Profile, which is available through Genova Diagnostics.

The Toxic Element Clearance Profile will identify aluminum, antimony, cadmium, lead, mercury, nickel, and other heavy metals that are toxic to breast tissue. For more information about testing, visit www.daniellachace.com.

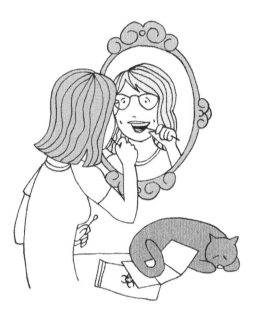

There are also genetic tests which identify the polymorphisms that hinder heavy metal clearance from our bodies. Genova Diagnostics offers the DetoxiGenomic Profile which is a simple buccal (cheek) swab test which only requires a cotton swab to be gently swiped on the inside of the mouth to collect a few cells for genetic testing.

Heavy Metal Reduction
Minerals provide protection from heavy metals, and studies have found that zinc, selenium, and iodine help reduce metal load in

the body. The ability of minerals to provide protection from metals makes them vital to prevention as well as treatment.

Sulfur nutrients that are found in brassica and allium vegetables as well supplements containing L-Methionine and N-acetyl cysteine (NAC) are effective at reducing the load of metals in the body through methylation. These nutrients are especially important for those who have a genetic weakness for clearance of metals. For example, those who have a Cytochrome P450 polymorphism.

N-acetyl cysteine, glycine, and L-glutamic acid are all dietary supplements that our bodies use to make the important detoxification nutrient glutathione. Practitioners often prescribe these as part of a heavy metals detox. They each play a role in the synthesis of glutathione which is a powerful detoxification agent that supports the excretion of many toxins, including heavy metals. Not only does glutathione help us excrete heavy metals, but our own internal production of glutathione is impaired when we are exposed to heavy metals. Therefore, it is even more important that we support our glutathione intake and production for heavy metals cleansing (Egiebor et al., 2013).

Melatonin reduces the damage from xenoestrogens such as heavy metals on estrogen-dependent tumors. Melatonin tests are available to help determine whether you need to take melatonin supplements or support your own natural melatonin production. Nightly, deep sleep can increase melatonin production. See the Self Care chapter for more about how to support better sleep.

Our bodies naturally excrete heavy metals at various rates of effectiveness depending on several factors, including our genetics, hydration level, and nutrient status. We excrete metals via urine, stool, and even some in our fingernails and hair. By hydrating well, increasing dietary fiber, and exercising we can boost excretion to a degree. We also excrete metals via sweat, which is why many detox programs that target metals include periodic saunas or steams to stimulate sweating. Be sure to replace lost fluids and electrolytes after a sweat.

Rosemary, turmeric, and holy basil have all been found to help retard breast cancer growth and progression. Their ability to increase the production of enzymes that support the elimination of toxins is a primary reason that they are so effective in reducing breast cancer growth.

Polyaromatic Hydrocarbons (PAHs)

PAHs and polycyclic aromatic hydrocarbons and heterocyclic amines have been found to suppress the immune system and increase the risk of breast cancer.

Sources

Our exposure to PAHs comes from smoke and charred fats such as cigarettes, second hand smoke, BBQs, burnt toast, VOG (volcanic smog), and campfires and forest fires. Smoke from burning coal, oil, gas, or wood all release PAHs.

Avoid eating burnt foods and inhaling smoke of all kinds. Cigarette smoke contains not only PAHs but also high levels of cadmium, which is used to slow the burning of the cigarette paper.

Early exposure to PAHs appears to increase the risk for breast cancer development, making it especially important that young woman avoid exposure.

Genetic Risk

PAH exposure affects those with a genetic weakness for the clearance of these toxins. Those of us who have a polymorphism in our cytochrome P450 and CYP1A1 clearance pathways are at a much higher risk for breast cancer development (Ishibe et al., 1998). These genes code for the enzyme involved in the metabolism of PAHs. When we aren't making enough of the enzymes to break down PAHs and clear them from our bodies, we have prolonged exposure.

Detoxification of PAHs

Epidemiological evidence strongly suggests that consumption of dietary phytochemicals found in vegetables and fruit can remediate exposure to PAHs. Glucosinolates from brassica vegetables boost the enzymes that break down these carcinogens (Abdull et al., 2013).

PAHs as Xenoestrogens

Exposures to environmental pollutants such as PAHs and dioxins are considered major risk factors in premenopausal breast cancer development. Researchers have observed that multiple exposures to other xenoestrogens such as oral contraception compound the estrogen effects, increasing risk significantly (Bidgoli et al., 2011).

Nutrient Support for Detoxifying PAHs

- Glutathione precursors, e.g., NAC
- Antioxidants, e.g., quercetin

Recommended Foods

- Rosemary
- Turmeric
- Holy Basil

Heterocyclic Amines (HCAs)

PhIP (2-Amino-1-methyl-6-phenylimidazo[4,5-b]pyridine) is one of the most abundant heterocyclic amines (HCAs) in cooked meat.

PhIP is particularly damaging to breast cells and a known trigger of breast cancer. Most cancer-causing agents are involved in either the initiation stage of cancer, triggering the initial DNA mutation (like radiation), or in the development stage of cancer, promoting the acceleration of the tumor. But PhIP has been called a three strikes carcinogen because it causes DNA mutations (strike one), and promotes cancer growth (strike two), and increases cancer spread (strike three).

PhIP is formed from the reaction between meat proteins and sugar when combined with high temperatures, such as grilling and frying. PhIP has been found to directly activate estrogen receptors on human breast cancer cells. PhIP is also found in cigarette smoke, diesel fumes, and incinerator ash, but the highest levels in food are found in fried bacon, fish, and chicken.

PhIP is particularly carcinogenic when combined with other toxins but its toxic effects can be dramatically reduced by drinking green tea (Pluchino et al., 2014).

Parabens

Parabens are common chemicals linked to breast cancer that are widely used as antimicrobial (antibacterial and antifungal) and commonly used as preservatives in our food, medications, and personal care products (Błędzka et al., 2014).

Parabens are often used as preservatives in personal care products such as cosmetics, shampoos, lotions, soaps, conditioners, and antimicrobial medications. These compounds can be easily absorbed by ingestion as well as through our skin where they can act as carcinogens.

Studies have found that even small amounts stimulate growth of cancer and that their carcinogenic effects could be increased by combining multiple types of parabens (Charles et al., 2013). Due to our multiple exposure through food, personal care products, and medications, this could be a significant risk factor for those with hormone-sensitive cancers, those who are postmenopausal, and the young.

Parabens Exposure

Parabens have been used in so many products over the last fifty years that they have become ubiquitous and are detectable in wastewater, rivers, soil, and house dust. Parabens have also been detected in human tissues and urine samples and most recently in higher levels in the breast tissue of patients with breast cancer (Genuis et al., 2013).

Estrogenic Effects of Parabens

Parabens have similar structure to estrogen and progesterone which means they have the ability to stimulate the growth of hormone-receptor-positive breast cancer subtypes. These compounds are known as endocrine disruptors because they mimic hormones (Mervish et al., 2014). They have been found to increase the risk for development of breast cancer, thyroid dysfunction, allergies, and obesity.

Parabens such as methyl-, propyl-, and butylparaben have the ability to act like estrogen as well as progesterone, and stimulate receptor sites, which may trigger the development and progression of hormone-sensitive breast cancer types. Parabens can influence not only proliferation but also movement of cancer cells throughout the body and increase the aggressiveness of human breast cancer cells (Khanna et al., 2014).

Epigenetic Effect

Parabens also have an epigenetic effect as they have the ability to activate cancer genes (Wróbel et al., 2014).

Avoid Exposure

Parabens are among the most commonly used preservatives used to reduce bacterial and fungal growth in cosmetic products such as makeup, moisturizers, and hair care and shaving products.

Avoid products containing parabens, which may be listed in the ingredients as methylparaben, propylparaben, ethylparaben, butylparaben, and isobutylparaben. Each of these compounds may also be listed by their chemical components on labels. Spend a few minutes on the EWG.org website to get an idea of which type of products carry these compounds and how to avoid them in the future.

Phthalates

Bisphenol A (BPA), is a chemical produced in large quantities for use primarily in the production of polycarbonate plastics and epoxy resins. It is found in food packaging, particularly plastic containers, such as baby bottles, and reusable water bottles, and is also in the epoxy resin linings of cans. It leaches from the packaging into the food. BPA effects breast cancer by interfering with the action of genes that protect against breast cancer, acting as an endocrine disruptor and stimulating growth of breast cancer cells.

Phthalates are being studied as they are either known to or are likely to cause cancer. On top of their carcinogenic potential, they are also molecules that are structurally similar to hormones and mimic hormones and can disrupt endocrine communication.

Tufts University researchers have identified BPA as a mammary carcinogen. They discovered that when they exposed rats to doses of BPA comparable to those seen in humans, BPA acted as a mammary gland carcinogen.

Epigenetic Trigger

BPA has a hypomethylating effect that turns on genes that lead to breast cancer. BPA has now been identified as an epigenetic trigger of breast cancer. Short-term exposure triggers a reversible epigenetic effect, whereas chronic exposure to BPA could potentially cause a permanent change (Patterson et al., 2015). However, detoxification and removal of BPA from body tissues is showing promise in the reversal of its effects.

BPA has been found to affect signaling pathways that influence cell proliferation and migration in breast cancer cells and cancer-associated fibroblasts.

Studies have found that babies, even before they are born, are susceptible to the effects of BPA. Therefore it's very important for children's health that pregnant women avoid exposure. Fortunately, there are many BPA-free products for adults and babies on the market already.

BPA is an endocrine disrupter. It is a synthetic estrogen mimicker. Hormonal disruption or imbalance leads to infertility, sexual and gender identity problems, diabetes, and even cancer.

BPA exerts estrogen-like activity on estrogen receptors and is involved in the proliferative effects induced in both normal and tumor cells.

Exposure

Plastic are everywhere it seems, so we have all had exposure. Even the CDC reported in 2004 that BPA has appeared in the urine of over 90 percent of those tested.

Risk Group ER+

Those with ER+ cancer are more affected by phthalates and other estrogenic mimickers as these compounds can turn on breast cancer genes that have estrogen receptors.

BPA has been found to exert its estrogen-like activity on ER+ tissue, which leads to proliferation in both normal and tumor cells.

Risk Group BRCA1 and BRCA2

Xenoestrogens are endocrine disruptors that may contribute to the development of hormone-dependent breast cancers. BPA exposure causes alternations in human breast epithelial cells. This suggest that the breast tissue of women with BRCA1 or BRCA2 mutations could be more susceptible to the effects of BPA.

Risk Group IBC

HER2 is the human epidermal growth factor receptor and is found in inflammatory breast cancer, or IBC. BPA not only accelerates cell growth in breast cancer but can also reduce the effectiveness of some treatments.

Epigenetic Effect

BPA and phthalates are epigenetically toxic and interfere with signaling pathways, histone modification, and expression of non-coding RNAs (including microRNAs) by making DNA methylation changes in human breast epithelial cells. BPA can trigger benign tumors to become cancerous and stimulate the growth and spread of existing breast cancer cells and tissues.

Determining Risk

Current research is focused around biomonitoring data in an effort to determine who is most at risk due to either exposure or genetic susceptibility. Until we know more, it is safest to take the cautionary approach and reduce exposure to phthalates as much as possible.

Reduce Exposure

Replace plastic cups and bowls in your kitchen with glass or ceramics. Store food in glass containers rather than plastic.

Buy canned foods only if the cans are labeled *BPA-free*. Never microwave food in plastic containers. Even water bottles left in a car on a warm day can leach BPA into the water.

We are exposed to BPA through our food because it is used in much of our food packaging. Restaurants often store and heat food in plastic.

Heat-resistant glass containers and stainless steel pans are BPA-free. Many of the glass food storage containers have plastic lids, but the lids rarely come in contact with the food, so they are not a concern.

Sources of Contamination

BPA is used in most plastic bottles, the inner linings of beverage and food cans, inks for store receipts, printers, and paper money, and some cosmetics and clothing apparel.

Some foods leach more plastic than others. For example, acidic foods and liquids break down plastic containers, allowing more of the plastic material to migrate into the foods we eat. Also, foods that have had extended contact with plastic have higher levels of BPA contamination.

Other sources of phthalates include polyvinyl chloride (PVC) pipes that carry drinking water into our homes and styrene which is used to make Styrofoam.

BPA Detoxification

To boost our ability to clear phthalates and their metabolites from our bodies, we can support detoxification with nutrients and microbes. These increase clearance in several ways: by inhibiting binding sites so that these toxic compounds can't adhere in our cells as easily; by increasing the production of enzymes that break down toxins, helping them to be flushed out through our digestive and urinary tracts; and through methylation, which helps us flush them from our bodies.

Protective Foods

Nutrients found in foods and supplements offer protection from phthalates by interfering with their toxic effects on our endocrine systems. Foods contain compounds that reduce the negative epigenetic effects caused by phthalates. For example, dietary supplementation of a methyl donor like methylfolate folate can compensate for the hypomethylating effect of phthalates. Also, microbes from fermented foods increase methylation which reduces the chances of negative epigenetic stimulation.

Certain nutrients help reduce the amount of BPA in our bodies. These include:

- Naringenin-containing foods such as citrus fruits
- Microbe-rich foods such as kefir, kimchi, and cultured coconut milk
- Catechins, found in black, green, and white tea
- Melatonin foods (bananas and cherries)
- Quercetin from apples and onions
- Folate from nutritional yeast

To determine whether you have had significant exposure to phthalates, consider the sources. If you have been microwaving in plastics, drinking out of plastic water bottles, or eat in restaurants frequently, your risk is higher than someone who eats meals at home made from whole, unprocessed foods cooked in stainless steel. Unfortunately, a modern lifestyle is one that inherently involves exposure to phthalates.

Laboratory tests are available that screen for various phthalate metabolites. Genova Diagnostics offers a Phthalates & Parabens Profile, which is a simple urine test. Many integrative oncology practitioners carry these tests in their offices, or they will send the test kits directly to your home. A urine sample is shipped to the lab and the results are sent to your practitioner's office so they can interpret the results for you.

Quality Supplements

A few high-quality supplement brands that I use in my office and highly recommend are Klaire, Integrative Therapeutics, Vital Nutrients, and Thorne Research.

Supplement Support

A few specific nutrients have been found to enhance excretion of phthalates and reduce their impact on the breast tissue. These are recommendations that you might discuss with you practitioner to determine the best program for you:

- Fractionated Pectin Powder (Thorne Research)
- Naringenin (Aura Cacia essential citrus oils)
- Quercetin (Quercenase from Thorne Research)
- Melatonin
- Folate (400 mcg. in methyl form rather than folic acid)
- Lysine
- Vitamin C (ascorbic acid)
- Citrus Bioflavonoid Complex

■ STRATEGY: DETOXIFICATION CHAPTER

Be aware of the toxins that affect breast cancer and the exposures that are most likely for you. Consider your home and work environment as well as your diet, and review the sources of contamination for each toxin. Eliminate toxins from your diet as much as possible. Replace toxic products such as lotions, cleaning supplies, and kitchen tools with non-toxic alternatives.

CHECKLIST

- Ask your doctor about SNP tests that check for polymorphisms that effect toxin clearance.
- Consider your past and current exposure to toxins such as heavy metals, parabens, phthalates and bromine. Order test kits, complete the collections (most of the kits require a urine sample) and send the samples in to the lab.
- When you receive your test results, consider nutrient supplementation to remediate the toxins.

For more support locating a physician, finding these tests, and keeping informed about nutrients that help specific subtypes, visit www.daniellachace.com.

Chapter Four

NUTRITION

In my clinical practice over the last two decades, I've seen the profound effects that nutrition has on disease development and reversal. More recently, nutrition studies from around the globe have changed the way we think about nutrition in disease management. Nutrition was once thought of as an adjuvant part of cancer care, only playing a supporting role in prevention. However, large-scale clinical trials have proven that food nutrients are necessary for healing and should be included in every treatment plan.

A nutrient-dense diet infuses our bodies with a constant supply of cofactors needed for proper function. Nutrients support our basic needs, such as sustained energy, brain fuel, hormone production, and digestion. They are also needed for more specific processes, including cell turnover, detoxification, immune function, and apoptosis, which is cancer cell destruction.

We need to take in nutrients consistently or we can develop deficiencies. When nutrient deficiencies go unaddressed, we limit the ability of our biological systems to function optimally. Nutrients not only support these key areas of health, but they also are cofactors in the removal of toxins and epigenetic management, and prevent secondary issues such as inflammation and other side effects of the cancer and its treatment.

A recent study suggests that women who eat lots of fruit, vegetables, and legumes and minimize red meat, salt, and processed carbohydrates may lower their odds of developing estrogen-receptor-negative breast cancer, which accounts for about a quarter of all breast cancers. Another study published in the *American Journal of Epidemiology* found that the likelihood of the cancer was 20 percent less when women followed a healthy diet.

A poor diet based on processed and packaged foods that are high in sugar and fat provide little nutritional value and drive the growth of breast cancer cells. Food quality varies dramatically as some foods have been so highly processed that they are devoid of nutrients and are laden with chemicals, many of which are known carcinogens.

Processed foods not only fall short of providing the necessary nutrients, but they also deliver unhealthy components, such as BPA from plastic food packaging, which drive the growth of cancer. Conversely, a nutritious diet can directly reduce the development, growth, and spread of breast cancer cells. Organic foods have been found to have a higher nutrient content and are free of agricultural chemicals. Many agricultural pesticides have been found to add to the risk of breast cancer and directly disrupt multiple metabolic pathways, which can prevent the body from properly defending itself against cellular mutations that lead to cancer.

To avoid exposure to these carcinogens, look for the USDA Organic label, as organic certification forbids the use of chemical pesticides or herbicides on plant foods for human consumption. To learn about which foods have the least contamination and which are most heavily sprayed, visit www.ewg.org.

Aim for the highest quality foods available, which means those that are organic, unprocessed, and as fresh as possible.

A nutrient-dense diet can provide the level of nutrients we need for maintenance. However, whole foods may not contain enough of specific nutrients needed to reverse a deficiency. For example, a vitamin D deficiency requires a high-dose supplement for several weeks to increase blood levels to a healthy level, after which a whole foods diet is sufficient to maintain a healthy level.

Dietary Goals

Avoid simple carbohydrates
Avoid alcohol
Avoid processed foods
Avoid red meat and dairy products
Avoid trans fat, saturated fat, and animal fat
Maintain proper hydration
Increase vegetables, including herbs and legumes
Increase plant foods
Increase fiber

Supporting Digestion

Our digestive processes are affected by a state of stress, which can reduce the quantity of enzymes and other digestive fluids produced by our bodies. When we don't have sufficient digestion, we don't properly metabolize our food or absorb the nutrients from that food. You may need to take digestive enzymes or probiotics to boost metabolism of food nutrients.

Our gut flora support digestion and often need to be replenished with fermented foods or probiotic supplements. Also, if your digestion is hindered, you may temporarily need to supplement with digestive enzymes.

If you are experiencing nausea, stomach cramps, or excess gas or bloating, you may benefit from seeing a nutritionist for guidance in improving your digestion.

The link between specific food nutrients and their intervention in the development of breast cancer has been well studied, clearly showing the benefits for the following foods.

Servings Per Day of Power Food Groups

Serving suggestions that guide the number
of servings to eat each day from each food group below, are provided.

Taste test foods from each category such as Allium Family Vegetables or Herbs and choose a few that you like such as onions and basil. Then try to incorporate them into your daily diet to give your body a daily infusion of their nutrients.

When you add up servings, this looks like a lot of food to eat daily, but there is overlap in food groups. For example, legumes provide protein, carbs, and flavonols, and legumes provides protein and essential fatty acids.

Daily Diet Sample Menu

A typical day may include the following and cover all categories:

- Breakfast: One half cup steel-cut oats, three tablespoons toasted Chia Seed, one citrus fruit, and a cup of green tea.
- Snack: A smoothie made with berries, cultured coconut milk, chia seed, and a peach.
- Lunch: Spinach salad, black beans, broccoli, and garlic dressing, and a cup of green tea.
- Snack: Hummus and cherry tomatoes on crackers with a cup of green tea.
- Dinner: Roasted brassica vegetables and tempeh with quinoa, avocado, and pesto.
- Dessert: Popcorn with nutritional yeast and Tuscan spice mix.

Power Food Groups

The following list was created based on research that found that daily intake of these food groups provides enough nutrients to affect breast cancer when eaten in concentrations and daily.

The serving sizes have been determined based on the amount fed to subjects daily in intervention studies. Of course, we still benefit from eating these foods occasionally but studies suggest that eating them daily maximizes their benefits.

Power Food Group Servings Per Day

Fats
    2 tablespoons oil (e.g., olive, flax, or nut oil)
    2 tablespoons seeds (e.g., chia or hemp)

Fluids
    6 cups water (e.g., filtered water)
    2 cups tea (e.g., green tea)

Fruit
    1 citrus fruit (e.g., mandarin orange)
    ½ cup carotenoid-rich foods (e.g., apricot or tomato sauce)
    ½ cup berries (e.g., wild blueberries)

Protein Foods
    60–120 grams per day from plant foods primarily

Vegetables
    1 cup greens (e.g., spinach or kale)
    1 cup brassica vegetables (e.g., broccoli or cauliflower)
    1 cup fresh herbs (e.g., basil leaves or cilantro)
    ½ cup cooked legumes (e.g., black beans or lentils)
    ½ cup fermented foods (e.g., sauerkraut)
    ½ cup allium vegetables (e.g., onions)
    1 tablespoon dried herbs (e.g., rosemary)
    1 teaspoon dried spices (e.g., turmeric)

Whole Grains
    1 cup lignan-rich grain (e.g., oats, barley, spelt, or rye)

Carbohydrates

Carbohydrates are one of the main macro-nutrient categories along with protein and fat. Food sources include whole grains, beans, peas, nuts, seeds, vegetables, and fruits.

Scientists emphasize that many risk factors for breast cancer are controllable. An overall poor diet, one that is high in sugar and fat while also low in fiber and nutrients, is responsible for one-third of all breast cancers and a driver of triple negative cancers. A high intake of refined carbohydrates is associated with increased breast cancer incidence.

According to a study published in the *American Journal of Clinical Nutrition*, a higher-fiber diet could lower breast cancer risk. Researchers found that for every ten grams of added fiber daily, which equals about one-half to one cup of beans, breast cancer risk decreased by 7 percent. The findings are based on ten studies involving more than 710,000 people over seven to eighteen years. Other high-fiber foods include vegetables, whole grains, and lentils.

A diet rich in complex carbs and low in simple carbohydrates is linked to reduced cases of breast cancer. Carbohydrates in their unrefined form are considered complex as opposed to simple or refined. Complex carbs are rich in natural soluble and insoluble fiber.

High blood sugar, or hyperglycemia, is the result of intake of more sugar than our bodies can metabolize at one time. Sugar in the blood causes damage to cells and, when uncontrolled, leads to nerve damage. High intake of sugar suppresses the immune system and white blood cell production while feeding cancer growth. High blood sugar also provides food for unhealthy microbial growth, such as fungi (candida) and unhealthy bacteria. Sugar also poses a higher risk for premenopausal than for postmenopausal breast cancer.

The uptake of sugar in malignant cells can increase the development of cancer and has an epigenetic effect on nonmalignant human breast cells leading to increased growth. Therefore, avoiding dietary sugar and maintaining a high level of protein and fiber intake are primary strategic goals in cancer recovery.

Hyperglycemia is common in cancer patients but can be reversed through diet, nutrients, and simple lifestyle changes. Increase plant foods that are rich in fiber, protein, and water, while reducing simple carbohydrates (especially sugar) and also exercising and getting adequate sleep.

Hyperglycemia has been linked to causing vitamin C deficiency. Maintaining optimal levels of ascorbic acid (vitamin C) is important for immune function. Higher levels of blood glucose appear to decrease not only blood levels but also cellular stores of ascorbic acid.

Protein

Protein, along with carbohydrate and fat, is one of the three macro-nutrients we need for good health. Adequate protein intake throughout our lifetime facilitates the growth, repair, and maintenance of every cell in our bodies.

When we eat food that contains protein, our digestive system breaks it down into amino acids, which are in turn used by our bodies for a multitude of tasks. Protein facilitates water balance, is a source of heat and energy, assists with disease resistance and cell repair, helps maintain blood sugar levels, fights fatigue, and is necessary for building and maintaining lean body mass, connective tissues, red blood cells, and enzymes.

Generally, the average diet provides adequate protein; however, when healing from treatments, protein requirements increase. It is important to be aware of protein sources and to include these foods at every meal and snack.

When we are at our healthiest, we need approximately 50 to 100 grams of protein per day depending on our life stage and activity level. While healing from cancer, we need approximately 65 to 125 grams of protein per day.

Protein Sources

Whole, organic plant foods are ideal. Beans, peas, lentils, nuts, and seeds are rich sources of protein that also provide fiber as well as anticancer phytochemicals. Plant foods are also naturally free of cholesterol.

Protein Chart

PORTION SIZE	FOOD	PROTEIN (grams)
3 ounces	Almonds	18
3 ounces	Sunflower seeds	15
3 ounces	Pumpkin seeds	15
2 tablespoons	Pea protein powder	14
½ cup	Oats	14
3 ounces	Cashews	13
2 tablespoons	Rice protein powder	11
½ cup	Black beans	11
½ cup	Chickpeas	10
½ cup	Lima beans	8
½ cup	Split peas	8
½ cup	Lentils	8
½ cup	Red beans	8
½ cup	Pinto beans	8
2 tablespoons	Almond butter	7
2 tablespoons	Chia seed	6
2 tablespoons	Hulled hemp seed	5
1 tablespoon	Peanut butter	4
½ cup	Green peas	4

Animal foods, on the other hand, can be high in saturated fat and cholesterol and contain almost no fiber. Animal foods also contain varying levels of hormones, which should be avoided by those with hormone-sensitive cancers. Saturated fats from animal foods have been found to increase breast cancer risk and growth. Animal fats, in general, should be minimized as they may contain animal hormones and cholesterol and contribute to body fat weight. Body fat cells produce estrogen that can stimulate breast cancer growth.

Dairy foods and red meat should be avoided due to their potential hormone and saturated fat content. This is especially true for those with hormone-sensitive cancers, as animal foods not only naturally contain hormones, but may also contain synthetic hormones (e.g., bovine growth hormone) and antibiotics, which are commonly used in dairy cows.

Quality Protein Foods

Excellent sources of plant protein include chia seed and hulled hemp seed as they are devoid of hormones and high in protein, essential fatty acids, and fiber. Chia and hemp are rich in omega-3 fatty acids, which not only reduce cancer growth, but also are anti-inflammatory. Reducing inflammation is important, as evidence suggests that inflammation may cause a majority of the fatigue felt during and after treatment.

Vegan, organic protein powders are easy to digest and can be added to smoothies, and cereal or baked into protein bars or cookies. They are often made from peas, rice, hemp, or chia.

- Legumes: Beans, peas, and lentils are vegan and rich in protein and fiber.
- Seeds, Nuts, and Nut Butters: Seeds, nuts, and nut butters are high in protein and rich in monounsaturated fatty acids.

Caloric Needs

Each day we need to make sure that we meet our minimal calorie requirement or our bodies will use the protein we eat for energy rather than to support our essential body functions. Ask your nutritionist to calculate your caloric needs.

Fats

There are several important distinctions when choosing dietary fats as some are harmful, such as charred broiled red meat due to their ability to trigger breast cancer growth.

Fats to avoid are those that are highly processed (hydrogenated oils), those that are high in omega-6 fatty acids (soy oil), those that have been heated to high temperatures (frying oil), and saturated and hormone-laden fats from animal foods.

A high-fat diet increases the risk of the most common forms of breast cancer by 20 percent. We've known for a long time that there is a strong link between cancer development and saturated fat that comes from butter, red meat, and dairy products. Heavy consumption of saturated fat was found to have an even bigger impact, raising the risk of hormone-sensitive breast cancer by 28 percent.

Trans Fats and Cancer

Trans fats are linked to higher rates of breast cancer. In a European study, the concentration of trans fats stored in body fat was associated with a greater incidence of breast cancer. Some trans fats have been structurally altered by a process called hydrogenation, which turns a liquid oil into a solid spread at room temperature, but trans fats are linked to higher rates of breast cancer. Look for monounsaturated fats for cooking, such as olive oil. Research suggests that this may be especially important to reduce breast cancer risk in those who are postmenopausal.

Omega-3 and Breast Cancer

Rich sources of omega-3 fatty acids include chia seed, hemp seed, and algae derived oil supplements. Studies have found that post-menopausal women who eat a diet high in fish containing omega-3 fatty acids have lower rates of breast cancer.

The omega three fatty acids are also called n-3 polyunsaturated fatty acids (n-3 PUFAs). PUFAs include eicosapentaenoic acid (EPA) and docosahexaenoic acid (DHA) which each exert anti-cancer effects and DHA increases the effectiveness of chemotherapy by increasing the sensitivity of tumors to the treatment.

Fish meat and fish oils bioaccumulate toxins such as mercury. Large fish are higher up the food chain and carry a heavier burden of toxins from the smaller fish they have eaten.

It is well established that omega-3 fatty acids can inhibit the growth of cancer cells. However, most diets are high in omega-6 fatty acids, while falling short of the recommended omega-3 fatty acid concentrations. Diets high in omega-6 fatty acids that do not also contain adequate amounts of omega-3 fatty acids are likely to increase breast cancer risk. Damaging omega-6 foods include corn oil, soy oils, and processed foods, and healthful omega-3 foods include, walnuts, and flaxseed. Flaxseed is such a rich source of omega-3 fatty acids that just 25 grams of flaxseed daily has been found to reduce growth of breast cancer cells. A recent animal study found that mice fed walnuts had significantly fewer breast tumors than the control group, which may be due to their omega-3 fatty acids and tocopherols (Hardman, 2014).

Omega-3 and TNBC

Omega-3 fatty acids not only inhibit the growth of breast cancer cells but also induce apoptosis. This inhibitory effect was found to be even more pronounced on triple negative breast cancer cells.

Excess omega-6 fatty acids may be particularly damaging for those who have a predisposition to metabolize them into higher levels of pro-inflammatory substances, based on genetic variability.

One difference in the way our bodies use omega-6 versus omega-3 fatty acids is how they regulate inflammation in our bodies. Omega-6 fatty acids promote inflammation while omega-3 fatty acids are converted almost exclusively into anti-inflammatory compounds. Thus, a diet high in omega-6 and low omega-3 is generally pro-inflammatory. This is a significant consideration as chronic inflammation plays an important role in the development and growth of breast cancer as well as its accompanying fatigue (Alfano et al., 2012).

Omega-6 fatty acids are partially converted enzymatically into arachidonic acid, an essential but inflammation-promoting eicosanoid. The enzyme levels influencing this conversion vary with genetic inheritance. Genetic variations responsible for higher enzyme levels of the fatty acid, desaturase, for example, are much more common in people of African than of European ancestry. The implications could be profound, since African and African-American women are at higher risk of more aggressive and hormone-receptor-negative tumors.

Omega-3 Fatty Acids

Portion Size	Food	Omega-3 Fatty Acids (grams)
1 tablespoon	Flaxseed oil	8
2 tablespoons	Chia seed	5
2 tablespoons	Flaxseed	3
2 tablespoons	Hulled hemp seed	3
¼ cup	Walnuts	3
1 tablespoon	Walnut oil	1
1 tablespoon	Extra virgin olive oil	1

The 5-lipoxygenase enzyme converts arachidonic acid to various inflammatory mediators called leukotrienes. The 5-lipoxygenase pathway has been implicated in carcinogenesis and tumor progression in breast cancer. A particular polymorphism responsible for levels of this enzyme increases risk for breast cancer only if the diet contains high levels of linoleic acid, the most prominent omega-6 polyunsaturated fatty acid.

Power Nutrient Groups

Two nutrient groups that play a central role in the healing of breast cancer include carotenoids and flavonols.

Carotenoids

Carotenoids are colorful, cancer-protective nutrients synthesized by plants, algae, and photosynthetic bacteria. They give many fruits and vegetables their distinctive yellow, orange, or red colors.

Carotenoids are divided into two classes, carotenes (alpha-carotene, beta-carotene, and lycopene) and xanthophylls (beta-cryptoxanthin, lutein, and zeaxanthin).

Carotenoids intervene in the development of breast cancer and reduce invasiveness of existing cells (Mignone et al., 2009). Many studies have found that women who eat plenty of carotenoid-rich foods have lower rates of breast cancer.

Prevention of Recurrence

Increasing fruit and vegetable intake can reduce the likelihood not just of breast cancer development, but of recurrence. In a study of over 1,500 women previously treated for early-stage breast cancer, those with the highest plasma carotenoid concentrations had the lowest rates of breast cancer recurrence, thanks to their fruit and vegetable intake.

When we eat carotenoid-rich vegetables frequently, we increase and maintain our serum (blood) concentration. Five servings of carotenoid-rich fruits and vegetables each day is enough to maintain these protective levels. Studies using serum measures of carotenoids found a significant protective association against breast cancer (Pouchieu et al., 2014). Women who have high mammographic density (areas of dense breast tissue) but who also have high blood carotenoid levels have been shown to have a 40–50 percent lower risk for developing breast cancer. This finding indicates that carotenoids in the diet can lower breast cancer risk almost by half, even in women who have a higher risk.

Also, those who already have breast cancer are found to have a better outcome when their blood levels of carotenoids are higher. The Women's Healthy Eating and Living (WHEL) intervention study showed improved prognosis after breast cancer diagnosis in individuals with the highest baseline levels of carotenoids.

Some Carotenoids Became Vitamin A

Alpha-carotene, beta-carotene, and beta-cryptoxanthin are also provitamin-A carotenoids, meaning they can be converted by the body to retinol (a vitamin A precursor). Vitamin A and retinol help boost the immune system.

Carotenoid Act as Antioxidants

Alpha-carotene, found in orange-colored vegetables and fruits, is most strongly associated with lower levels of cellular oxidation. All of the carotenoids are potent antioxidants, meaning that they bind to free radicals. Free radicals are atoms or molecules that cause damage by reacting with fats and proteins in cell membranes and genetic material. This reaction is called oxidation. It can damage cells and cause cancerous changes. When an antioxidant attaches to a free radical, it becomes impossible for the free radical to react with, or oxidize, other molecules. In this way, antioxidants may protect against the development of cancer.

Cell Division Support

Also, carotenoids help maintain cell differentiation. Cell differentiation is the ability of cells in the body to develop differently and have different functions. This ability is often absent in cancer cells and may be a reason for their uncontrolled growth. Beta-carotene, one of the major carotenoids, may be particularly important because it is converted to vitamin A. Vitamin A is in turn converted to retinoic acid, which tends to reduce cellular proliferation, encourage cellular differentiation, and inhibit angiogenesis.

Cellular Communication

Carotenoids also act as epigenetic (gene-modifying) nutrients that facilitate intercellular communication by increasing gene expression.

Apoptosis

Carotenoids also have the ability to induce apoptosis (cell death) in cancer cells (Bolhassani et al., 2015). Tumors occur because the fast-growing cancer cells do not die off like normal cells do. Many studies have shown that carotenoids increase the rate of apoptosis in cancer cells, which reduces cancerous cells and tumor size. Lycopene and beta-carotene, in particular, have been shown to induce apoptosis in breast cancer cells (Gloria et al., 2014).

Flavonols and Breast Cancer

Flavonols are found in fruits, vegetables, beans, peas, and lentils are important anticancer nutrients. Flavonols from foods rather than supplements are more effective. Healthy levels of gut flora help us digest these nutrients whether from food or supplements.

Flavonols act as antioxidants providing anti-inflammatory and antimicrobial benefits. Specifically, they have been found to arrest cell cycles as well as inhibit growth and spread of breast cancer

Carotenoid-Rich Foods

Alpha-carotene
  Asparagus
  Arugula
  Bananas
  Beans
  Beets
  Cabbage
  Carrots
  Cilantro
  Collard greens and
      other dark
      leafy greens
  Peas
  Pumpkin
  Red bell peppers
  Tangerines
  Tomatoes
  Winter squash
Beta-carotene
  Apricots
  Arugula
  Asparagus
  Bananas
  Broccoli
  Cantaloupe
  Carrots
  Chinese cabbage
  Chives
  Kale

Grapefruit
Mangoes
Peas
Pumpkin
Spinach
Turnip greens
Sweet potatoes
Winter squash
Beta-cryptoxanthin
  Apricots
  Beets
  Cantaloupe
  Carrots
  Chili powder
  Corn
  Honeydew melons
  Nectarines
  Oranges
  Papaya
  Paprika
  Peaches
  Pumpkin
  Red bell peppers
  Tangerines
  Watermelon
Lutein and zeaxanthin
  Beets
  Broccoli
  Brussels sprouts

Collard greens
Corn
Green beans
Kale
Melons
Mustard greens
Oranges
Peas
Pumpkin
Spinach
Summer squash
Turnip greens
Winter squash
Lycopene
  Apricots
  Asparagus
  Beets
  Carrots
  Guavas
  Mango
  Papaya
  Pink grapefruit
  Red or purple
      cabbage
  Red bell peppers
  Sweet red peppers
  Tomatoes
  Watermelon

cells in laboratory studies. Flavonols also directly support apoptosis (Lea, 2015).

Quercetin is a major flavonoid compound with potential anti-metastatic effects as it has been found to inhibit invasion and migration of cancer cells in stress-related breast cancer. Quercetin may function by controlling signaling of adrenaline and noradrenaline, which are released from the adrenal glands during exposure to stress.

Ellagic acid is a dietary flavonoid polyphenol which is present in abundance in pomegranate, muscadine grapes, walnuts, and strawberries, has been shown to inhibit proliferation and induce apoptosis in breast cancer cells (Chen et al., 2015).

Power Food Groups

Several food groups that contain nutrients needed to support healing of breast cancer include allium vegetables, berries, brassica vegetables, citrus, herbs and spices, stone fruit, and tea.

Allium Vegetables
Alliums include garlic, leeks, onions, and scallions. These pungent plant foods contain concentrated amounts of antiviral and antitumor compounds.

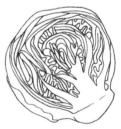

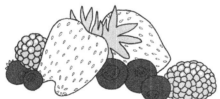

Berries
Berries include black chokeberries, black currants, blueberries, cherries, cranberries, grapes lingonberries, raspberries, and strawber-

ries. They contain antioxidants called anthocyanins that have been found to inhibit the growth and decrease the proliferation of breast cancer cells. Researchers believe the combination of carotenoids, anthocyanins, and high levels of vitamin C in berries have a synergistic effect, enhancing the benefits of each nutrient.

Brassica Vegetables

These hearty vegetables are also known as cruciferous or mustard family and include arugula, bok choy, broccoli, Brussels sprouts, cabbage, cauliflower, Chinese cabbage, collard greens, cress, horseradish, kale, kohlrabi, mustard greens, radish, rutabaga, turnips, wasabi, and watercress. Brassica vegetables contain powerful nutrients that have a direct affect on hormone regulation.

Citrus

Citrus fruits, such as oranges, tangerines, grapefruit, lemons, and limes contain nutrients that concentrate in the breast tissue and reduce breast cancer cell growth.

Herbs and Spices

Certain herbs and spices contain concentrated bioactives, including phenolic acids, flavonoids, tannins, stilbenes, curcuminoids, coumarins, lignans, and quinones. Herbs are the fragrant leaves of plants that contain nutrient-rich oils and include basil, holy basil, sage, and rosemary. Spices are made from the seeds and nuts of plants. Spices that have been studied for their anticancer properties include allspice, black pepper, caraway, cardamom, cinnamon, cloves, cumin, mustard, nutmeg, rosemary, saffron, turmeric, and vanilla.

Daily intake of fresh and dried herbs and spices may help neutralize free radicals and protect cells from the oxidative stress that can lead to cancerous mutations.

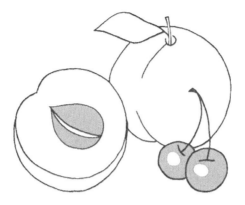

Stone Fruit

Stone fruits include apricots, figs, peaches, plums, prunes, and nectarines. They contain antioxidant carotenoids that can reduce precancerous cell changes, which have the potential to become breast tumors.

Tea

Green, black and white tea are all made from the buds and leaves of the Camellia sinensis plant and contain polyphenol antioxidants. Green tea is made when the leaves are minimally oxidized and white tea has the additional fine silvery-white hairs from the unopened buds of the tea plant which is what makes the tea look white or pale yellow.

■ STRATEGY: NUTRITION CHAPTER

Use the Foods to Avoid list to guide you in removing unhealthy foods from your kitchen. Review the Daily Diet Sample Menu and consider how you will create a menu for yourself based on the Foods to Eat list. Aim for the recommended number of servings per day for each food category. Once you have chosen the foods that you will eat each day, make a grocery list that you can use each week.

CHECKLIST

- Go through your cupboards and your refrigerator and replace unhealthy foods (such as those from the Foods to Avoid list in the next chapter) with healthier alternatives.
- Incorporate as many of the foods on the Foods to Eat list (see next chapter) into your diet as possible.
- Talk to your doctor or nutritionist about having your vitamin, mineral, and amino acid levels tested.
- Supplement with nutrients to correct any nutrient deficiencies.

For more support in locating a nutritionist, finding these tests, and keeping informed about nutrients that help specific subtypes, visit www.daniellachace.com.

FOODS TO EAT

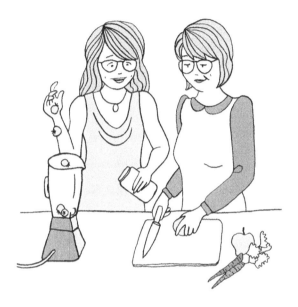

These foods are recommended because they provide nutrients that target breast cancer. However, it is important to keep in mind that food nutrients that support the prevention and healing of breast cancer need to be a part of your daily diet to provide medicinal benefit. Consistent ingestion of these nutrients can exert biological effects on the processes that hinder cancer progression.

Foods to Eat

Research has demonstrated that specific foods contain nutrients that provide a direct benefit in breast cancer treatment and prevention. Foods that have not yet been well-studied or were found to have negligible effects on breast cancer have not been included in this list.

Allium Vegetables
    Garlic
    Leeks
    Onions
    Scallions
Apples
Bananas
Beans
Beets
Bell Peppers
Berries
    Blueberries
    Cherries
    Cranberries
    Black currants
    Black chokeberries
    Grapes
    Lingonberries
    Marionberries
    Raspberries
    Strawberries
    Tart cherries
Brassica Vegetables
    Arugula
    Bok choy
    Broccoli
    Brussels sprouts
    Cabbage
    Cauliflowers
    Chinese cabbage
    Collard greens
    Horseradish
    Kale
    Kohlrabi
    Mustard greens
    Radishes
    Rutabagas
    Sauerkraut
    Turnips
    Wasabi
    Watercress

Carrots
Celery
Citrus Fruits
    Grapefruit
    Lemons
    Limes
    Oranges
    Tangerines
Cocoa
Coffee
Coconut Milk
    Coconut milk, unsweetened
    Cultured coconut milk
Cucumber
Ginger
Greens
    Arugula
    Collard greens
    Dandelion greens
    Kale
    Lettuce
    Mustard greens
    Romaine lettuce
    Spinach
    Swiss chard
Guava
Herbs
    Basil
    Cilantro
    Holy basil
    Rosemary
    Sage
    Thyme
Legumes
    Black beans
    Garbanzo beans
    Lentils
    Navy beans
    Peanuts
    Peas
    Pinto beans

Mangoes
Melons
    Cantaloupe
    Honeydew
    Muskmelon
    Watermelon
Mustard
Nutritional Yeast
Nuts and Seeds
    Almonds
    Brazil nuts
    Cashews
    Chia seed
    Flaxseed
    Hazelnuts
    Hemp seed
    Pecans
    Pumpkin seeds
    Sesame seeds
    Sunflower seeds
    Walnuts
Oils
    Avocado oil
    Coconut oil
    Olive oil
    Peanut oil
    Sesame oil
    Walnut oil
Papaya
Pineapple
Pomegranate
Potatoes
    Purple potatoes
    Sweet potatoes
    Yams
    Yukon Gold
Protein Powder
    Chia protein powder
    Hemp protein powder
    Pea protein powder
    Rice protein powder
Salt
Spices
    Allspice
    Black Cumin
    Black pepper
    Caraway
    Cardamom

    Cinnamon
    Cumin
    Ginger
    Mustard
    Nutmeg
    Paprika
    Rosemary
    Saffron
    Turmeric
    Vanilla beans
    Vanilla extract
Squash
    Acorn squash
    Buttercup
    Butternut
    Crookneck
    Pumpkin
    Summer squash
    Winter squash
    Zucchini
Stone Fruits
    Apricots
    Peaches
    Plums
    Nectarines
Sweeteners
    Erythritol
    Coconut fiber
    Mannitol
    Stevia
    Xylitol
Tea
    Herbal tea
    Green tea
    White tea
Tomatoes
Vinegar
Water
Wheatgrass
Whole Grains
    Barley
    Kamut
    Oats
    Quinoa
    Rice
    Rye
    Spelt
    Teff

For example, food nutrients have been found to:

- Induce apoptosis
- Inhibit migration of cancer cells
- Reduce angiogenesis
- Support white blood cell production
- Reduce inflammation
- Improve immune response
- Reduce breast cancer cell growth
- Inhibit proliferation of cancer cells
- Decrease metastasis
- Inhibit microbial growth

Descriptions are provided for some of the more unusual ingredients, as well as information about where to find them in your local store or online.

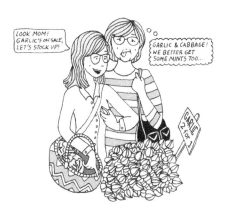

For definitions of any medical, technical, or nutrition terms, see the glossary of terms.

Allium Vegetables

Alliums include garlic, leeks, onions, and scallions. Garlic and its products all contain nutrients that fight breast cancer, including fresh garlic, garlic oil, dried garlic (flakes, powder, granules), and pills of aged garlic extract. Garlic provides diallyl trisulfide, which has the ability to induce apoptosis (Chandra-Kunal et al., 2013). Garlic also contains oleanolic acid or oleanic acid that reduces growth of breast cancer cells. Garlic supplements (aged garlic in capsules) were found to also arrest cell growth (Modem et al., 2012).

Onions contain oils that support immune function and help prevent viral, bacterial, and fungal infections.

Apples

Apples contain quercetin, a powerful antioxidant with proapoptotic effects against breast cancer cells. Apples also contain triterpene, which has proven antitumor action. Both triterpenes and quercetin reduce inflammation, improve immune response, and slow breast cancer cell growth. These nutrients are most prevalent in apple skins.

Fresh whole apples last for many weeks in a cool place, for instance the garage or in the crisper drawer of the refrigerator. Chopped apples can be stored in a glass-covered container for up to a week in the refrigerator. Applesauce contains fiber and many of the nutrients of fresh whole apples.

Organic, unfiltered apple juice also provides many of the breast cancer–fighting nutrients found in whole fruit. However, clear apple juice provides little benefit. Look for juice and sauce sold in glass containers to avoid the potential exposure to phthalates inherent in plastic bottles.

Fresh apple juice can be made at home with a juicer. Most blenders and food processors are powerful enough to blend whole apples with their skin intact.

Avocados

Avocados are a rich source of fiber and essential fatty acids such as gamma–linoleic acid (GLA), which confers anti-inflammatory and proapoptotic properties.

Bananas

Bananas provide electrolytes, alpha- and beta–carotene, and melatonin. They also contain oligofructose or oligosaccharides, a form of fiber that acts as a prebiotic and helps foster the growth of healthful bacteria in the gut. Bananas are also a rich source of dopamine, which can improve mood, sleep, and memory as well as acting as a powerful antioxidant. They also contain dietary melatonin, an antioxidant that reduces angiogenesis and triggers apoptosis of breast cancer cells.

Beans

Beans are large edible plant seeds. Common beans include green, kidney, lima, navy, pinto, black, soy, and garbanzo beans (chickpeas). Beans provide protein and both soluble and insoluble fiber. Fiber holds moisture in the intestines, which supports sustained hydration. Fiber also promotes the growth of probiotics, which help improve bowel health. Beans contain flavonols, which are antioxidants with anti-inflammatory, antimicrobial, and anticancer benefits. In a large study, higher intake of lentils and beans was associated with a lower incidence of breast cancer; the researchers concluded that this was due to the flavonol compounds found in these vegetables.

Beets

Beets are root vegetables that are usually red but may be orange, yellow, or even white. They can be eaten raw or cooked. Beets contain the carotenoid compounds alpha-carotene, beta-cryptoxanthin, lycopene, lutein, and zeaxanthin. These compounds neutralize free radicals and protect cells from the oxidative stress that can lead to cancerous mutations. Women who consume more carotenoid-rich fruits and vegetables have higher blood levels of carotenoids. High blood carotenoid levels are associated with a 40–50 percent lower risk for breast cancer in women found to have high mammographic density.

Bell Peppers

Red bell peppers are a rich source of vitamin C and the carotenoid lycopene. Studies have found that those who have the highest levels of carotenoids in their blood have the lowest risk for breast cancer. Beta-cryptoxanthin, beta-carotene, and lycopene provide protection against the development and growth of breast cancer cells.

Berries

Berries include blueberries, strawberries, cranberries, black currants, black chokeberries, lingonberries, cherries, raspberries, and grapes.

Berries contain nutrients that support breast cancer recovery including:

- Anthocyanins that may inhibit the growth of breast cancer cells
- Melatonin and vitamin C
- Cyanidin, delphinidin, kaempferol quercetin, ellagic acid, resveratrol, and pterostilbene that affect receptor pathways, reducing development of breast cancer cells and providing an epigenetic effect in turning off breast cancer genes
- Resveratrol, a stilbene that is anti-inflammatory, antimicrobial, and antiestrogenic

Brassica Vegetables

The Brassica or mustard family of vegetables includes arugula, bok choy, broccoli, Brussels sprouts, cabbage, cauliflower, Chinese cabbage, collard greens, horseradish, kale, kohlrabi, mustard greens, radish, rutabaga, turnips, wasabi, and watercress.

Brassica vegetables contain nutrients that support breast cancer recovery including:

- Indole-3-carbinol and diindolylmethane (DIM), which regulate sex hormone homeostasis
- The sulfur compounds glucosinolates and isothiocyanate which reduce excess estrogen
- Alpha- and beta-carotenes, and xanthophyll, which reduce oxidative stress and free radicals

Carrots

Carrots contain high amounts of antioxidant carotenoids, which can reduce precancerous cell changes that may lead to the formation of breast tumors. Scientists believe that alpha- and beta-carotenes act as cancer-preventative agents by reducing oxidative stress and free radicals in the body. A significant association exists between higher blood carotenoid levels and lower numbers of cell markers of oxidative stress. Alpha-carotene, found in orange-colored vegetables and fruits, provides the strongest antioxidant effects against cellular oxidation.

Celery
Celery contains carotenoids, which are associated with a significant reduction for risk of breast cancer in women who have high mammographic density.

Citrus Fruits
Oranges, lemons, limes, tangerines, and grapefruit contain nutrients that support breast cancer recovery. Citrus peel oil contains tangeretin, a nutrient compound known to have anticancer activities. Tangeretin-induced apoptosis has been observed in breast, colorectal, and lung cancers. Citrus peels also contain high levels of limonene, a lipophilic monoterpene that shows promise in studies for breast cancer prevention and growth inhibition.

The citrus flavonoids include hesperidin (a glycoside of the flavanone hesperetin), quercitrin, rutin (two glycosides of the flavonol quercetin), and the flavone tangeritin.

Citrus fruit, peel, and juices contain an antioxidant flavonoid called hesperidin that inhibits the growth and replication of breast cancer cells.

Grapefruit is rich in lycopene, an antioxidant which reduces the free radicals that lead to oxidative damage. Additionally, lycopene from grapefruit interferes with cancer cell growth and helps the body detoxify. Grapefruit also contains the flavonoids naringenin and nobiletin.

Cocoa
Cocoa, produced from the cocoa bean, is the main ingredient in all forms of chocolate.

Flavonoids exist naturally in unprocessed, unsweetened cocoa nibs and cocoa powder.

Pentameric procyanidin, a flavonoid found in cocoa, inhibits growth of human breast cancer cells. Cocoa also contains epicatechin, an antioxidant flavonol. The antioxidant and antiproliferative activity of theobroma cacao (cocoa) has a cytotoxic effect on cancer cells, but not in normal cells (Baharum et al., 2014).

Coffee
Coffee is a significant source of caffeine, a stimulant. Studies show that caffeine derivatives may help block cancer cells from forming or inhibit cancers from growing through apoptosis.

Coconut Milk
Coconut milk is the liquid that results when coconut meat is grated and pressed. It is commonly used as a milk alternative and in cooking. Cultured coconut milk contains probiotic organisms, such as Lactobacillus acidophilus, which has been found in laboratory studies to enhance the body's immune response against breast cancer.

Cucumbers
Cucurbaticins, the bitter substances in cucumbers, have an inhibitory effect on breast cancer cells and inflammation.

Ginger
Ginger comes from the root of the ginger plant. It is not technically a spice, although dried and powdered ginger can be found in the spices section of the grocery store. Ginger contains a compound called gingerol, which breaks down with heat, drying, or cooking into other compounds. One of these compounds, shogaol, has been shown to suppress cancer cell invasion and inflammation; it also displayed cytoprotective effects through modulation of signaling pathways (Gan et al., 2013). Fresh, raw ginger as well as cooked ginger provides benefits against breast cancer. Ginger also helps reduce chemotherapy-induced nausea.

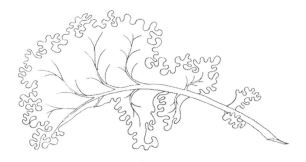

Greens

Arugula, kale, lettuce, spinach, turnip greens, parsley, and dandelion greens are rich sources of carotenoids and other nutrients that support breast cancer recovery.

Studies have repeatedly found that women who have higher levels of carotenoids in their blood from eating carotenoid-rich foods, have a lower risk for developing or experiencing a recurrence of breast cancer. In particular, lutein and zeaxanthin, both found in dark-green leafy vegetables, have been shown to provide protection against breast cancer.

Spinach contains bioactive glycolipid compounds that have an antitumor effect. Glycolipid compounds may inhibit the replication of many types of cancerous cells and reduce the size of tumors by inducing apoptosis in abnormal cells. Frequent intake of foods containing glycolipids, such as spinach, may help reduce tumor size due to these anticarcinogenic effects. Spinach is also an excellent source of carotenes.

Guava

Guava fruit is a good source of lycopene, an antioxidant that reduces the free radicals. Lycopene helps prevent oxidative damage, a precursor to abnormal cellular mutations that cause breast cancer. Guavas also contain carotenoids and polyphenols, two classes of antioxidants. Guavas that are red-orange have more polyphenols and carotenoids than the yellow-green ones.

Herbs

Herbs are the leaves of various plants used for flavor in cooking. Examples of herbs include basil, cilantro, rosemary, sage, thyme, and tulsi (holy basil).

Herbs contain nutrients that support breast cancer recovery, such as:

- Apigenin, a polyphenol antioxidant found in thyme and an anti-inflammatory against human breast cancer cells
- Carnosic acid, an antioxidant in rosemary that is a natural anti-inflammatory
- Oleanolic or oleanic acid found in holy basil that exhibits antitumor and antiviral properties
- Phenolic compounds which include phenolic acids, flavonoids, tannins, stilbenes, curcuminoids, coumarins, lignans, quinones, and others
- Rosmarinic acid, which is in both fresh and dried rosemary, rich sources of this natural phenolic compound

Legumes

Legumes are the fruits or seeds of plants in the Fabaceae family. They include beans, peas, lentils, and peanuts. Regular consumption of legumes is linked to lower breast cancer risk. Scientists believe this may be due to flavonol compounds found in these vegetables that provide a host of anti-inflammatory, antimicrobial, and anti-cancer mechanisms. Red peanut skin contains significant polyphenol content, including flavonoids.

Mangoes

Mangoes contain mangiferin, a bioactive xanthonoid, which is a natural plant polyphenol that has the ability to inhibit cancer and promote apoptosis (Matkowski et al., 2013). They are also an excellent source of beta-carotene, a powerful antioxidant.

Melons

Cantaloupe and honeydew melons are rich in alpha-carotene, beta-carotene, lutein, beta-cryptoxanthin, and zeaxanthin. These antioxidant compounds neutralize free radicals and protect cells from the oxidative stress that can lead to cancerous mutations.

Lycopene, an antioxidant found in watermelon, can reduce cancerous cells that lead to breast tumors.

Milk Alternatives

Dairy foods such as milk, butter, cheese, and ice cream should be avoided as they contain natural animal hormones and also may contain synthetic injected hormones such as bovine growth hormone, which increases hormone-sensitive cancer growth.

There are many milk alternatives that can be used in place of dairy milk, such as almond milk, coconut milk, hemp milk, and oat milk. They vary in their carbohydrate, fat, and calorie content. The plain varieties contain less sugar than the vanilla and chocolate flavored products.

Nutritional Yeast

Nutritional yeast contains ergosterol, a compound found to inhibit the growth of breast cancer cells, probably because of its antioxidant properties.

Interestingly, stored (rather than freshly prepared) ergosterol was more effective at inducing apoptosis in breast cancer cells in a laboratory study. This makes nutritional yeast a potentially more effective way to add ergosterol to your diet, rather than through active yeasts like Brewer's yeast.

Nuts and Seeds

Nuts and seeds include chia seed, flaxseeds, hemp seed, pumpkin seeds, almonds, Brazil nuts, cashews, hazelnuts, pecans, and walnuts.

Nuts and seeds are a source of beneficial lignans that may suppress the growth or spread of breast cancer cells by reducing the tumor-stimulating effects of circulating estrogen. The lignans, found in nuts and seeds (e.g., flax, chia, and sunflower seeds) reduce free estrogen.

Chia Seed—Chia seed comes from the Salvia hispanica plant, a South American member of the mint family. The seeds are an excellent source of fiber, protein, and cancer-protective omega-3 fatty acids, as well as calcium, magnesium, manganese, and phosphorus. Chia seed is also rich in antioxidants that help prevent cancer. A good way to incorporate these tiny seeds into your daily diet is to add them to smoothies. They can be used whole or ground in a coffee grinder to break down their husks which releases their oils and protein.

Flaxseed—Whole flaxseed and flaxseed oil are rich in omega-3 fatty acids. But they also contain phytoestrogens, which has made them a controversial food for estrogen-sensitive breast cancer patients. However, the discovery that their lignan content can counter the estrogen-mimicking effects has brought them back onto the list of recommended foods in the breast cancer diet. Whole flaxseeds contain higher levels of lignans than the oil, which makes them an even safer option.

Borage—Both borage oil and primrose oil have been found to reduce neuropathies and post-surgical numbness by improving nerve regeneration after surgery.

Hemp Seed—Hemp seed is rich in omega-3 fatty acids and protein. Hemp seed has been reported to have an antiproliferative effect on cancer cells, including aggressive breast cancers. These nourishing seeds contain cannabidiolic acid that inhibits the growth and spread of breast cancer cells (Takeda et al., 2012).

Hulled hemp seed is usually packaged without the seed's protective outer shell. This form is called hulled hemp seed, dehulled hemp seed, hemp hearts, or hemp nut. Hulled hemp seed has a sweet nutty flavor. It blends well in smoothies and is excellent in salads when toastved. It can be used in place of cheese in recipes.

Pumpkin Seeds—Pumpkin seeds are a rich source of dietary zinc, important for protection against cancer and for optimal immune function. Proper amounts of zinc are also necessary for the production of enzymes that digest food. Enzymes help the absorption of nutrients and protein, promoting overall health while reducing cancer risk.

Sesame Seeds—Sesame seeds are one of the richest food sources of lignans, compounds that have been found to reduce the growth of breast cancer cells. All nuts can be ground into a paste, just as peanuts are made into peanut butter. Ground sesame seeds are called tahini, which is a paste used in hummus and other lignan-rich dips and sauces.

Sunflower Seeds—Sunflower seeds are one of the richest dietary sources of beneficial lignans, which have been found to reduce the risk of breast cancer cell growth.

Walnuts—Walnuts and their oil are excellent sources of omega-3 fatty acids, selenium, phosphorous, magnesium, zinc, iron, and calcium. Walnuts and walnut oil also provide vitamins B1, B2, B3, and vitamin E.

Oils

Avocado Oil—Avocado oil can help your body absorb carotenoids, the anticancer compounds found in orange, yellow, and red vegetables.

Coconut Oil—Coconut oil provides healthful fats and antioxidants. One study reported that women being treated for breast cancer had fewer symptoms and a better quality of life when using a virgin coconut oil supplement daily.

Olive Oil—Olive oil contains monounsaturated fatty acids, which may help regulate genes involved in cancer and reduce cancer cell growth. Choose olive oil labeled extra virgin, which means it comes from the first press of the olives and no chemical solvents are used in the extraction of the oil. Extra virgin olive oil contains higher concentrations of nutrients, such as oleic acid, believed to regulate cancer-related oncogenes.

Peanut Oil—Peanuts have more antioxidants than many fruits. While they have not been studied for breast cancer, a ten-year study found that peanuts could reduce the risk of colon cancer. Peanuts also contain oleic acid, the healthy fat found in olive oil.

Sesame Oil—Sesame seeds contain lignans, compounds that have been shown to have anticancer effects.

Walnut Oil—Walnut oil is one of the best sources of omega-3 fatty acids, which have been proven to have anticancer effects.

Papaya
Papaya contains antioxidant carotenoids; higher carotenoid levels in the blood are linked to lower numbers of breast cancer cells. Laboratory studies have found that papaya extracts have significant antiproliferative and antineoplastic activities.

Pineapple
Pineapple, whether fresh, canned, or frozen, contains concentrated amounts of bromelain, an enzyme that has been found to promote apoptosis, particularly in breast cancer cells.

Pomegranate

Pomegranate seeds and juice contain polyphenols, which have been shown to reduce breast cancer cell growth. One of these polyphenols, ellagic acid, has been shown to kill cancer cells, stop tumor growth, and prevent carcinogens from binding to cell DNA. Pomegranate juice is being studied not only as a preventive agent but also for its effect as a selective estrogen receptor modulator for breast cancer.

Potatoes

Yellow, purple, white, and orange potatoes each have slightly different nutrient content. The yellow and orange forms of potatoes, especially sweet potatoes, contain carotenoids that have antioxidant effects. Purple sweet potatoes contain anthocyanins, molecules that have been shown to reduce cancer cell growth. Anthocyanins fight cancerous cells by inducing apoptosis, and also act as free radical scavengers.

Yams have healthy effects on sex hormones, lipids, and antioxidant levels, and may help prevent breast cancer in postmenopausal women.

Protein Powder

Many forms of protein powder are now available, including vegetable protein powders made from rice, peas, or hemp. Whey- or casein-based protein powders are made from dairy, so those who need to avoid dairy, such as those with ER+ or PR+ subtypes, should not use whey protein powders.

Salt

Salt is the common name for sodium chloride, a mineral necessary for proper functioning of the body. Use iodized salt, as it contains the mineral iodine and is one of the few food sources of iodine in the typical American diet.

Spices

Spices are made from the flavorful seeds and nuts of plants, and are primarily used for flavoring. Spices that have been studied for their anticancer properties include allspice, black pepper, caraway, cardamom, cinnamon, cloves, cumin, mustard, nutmeg, rosemary, saffron, turmeric, and vanilla.

These spices contain nutrients that support breast cancer recovery.

Allspice—Allspice provides eugenol, which has antioxidant and antimicrobial properties.

Black cumin—Black cumin seeds of nigella sativa contain thymoquinone, which has showed efficiency in killing cancer cells and retarding cell migration (Bhattacharya et al., 2015).

Black pepper—Black pepper contains piperine that can help regulate inflammation and also inhibit angiogenesis.

Caraway—Caraway reduces free radicals, lowers oxidative stress, and may also inhibit cancer cell growth.

Cardamom—Cardamom contains high amounts of limonene, a bioactive food component that concentrates in breast tissues and has chemopreventive and chemotherapeutic activities.

Cinnamon—Cinnamon is high in antioxidant polyphenols.

Cloves—Cloves are rich in antioxidants.

Cumin—Cumin contains thymoquinone, a compound reported to have antioxidant, antimicrobial, and anti-inflammatory properties, as well as the ability to suppress tumor growth.

Mustard—Mustard seeds are rich in glucosinolates and isothiocyanates, both of which are anti-inflammatory.

Saffron—Saffron has been shown in many studies to have strong anticancer qualities, both in preventing cancer from developing and inhibiting the growth of tumors.

Nutmeg—Nutmeg contains several lignans that have a cytotoxic effect against cancer cells.

Paprika—Paprika contains bioactive components that have been found to suppress the proliferation, invasion and migration of breast cancer cells.

Rosemary—Rosemary contains carnosol and rosmarinic acid, which have potent cytotoxicity action against breast cancer cells.

Turmeric—Turmeric is made from the cooked, ground-up rhizome of the turmeric plant. Turmeric contains high amounts of curcumin, a compound that has been shown to reduce insulin-like growth factor (IGF-1) in animal studies. Scientists believe that IGF may contribute to tumor growth by protecting cancerous cells from apoptosis.

Vanilla beans—Vanilla beans and vanilla extract contain vanillin, a polyphenol that has strong antioxidant and anticarcinogenic properties.

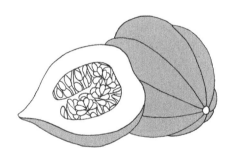

Squash

Pumpkin, acorn, buttercup, butternut, and turban winter squash contain carotenoids that can reduce precancerous cell changes that may lead to the formation of breast tumors. A significant association has been found between higher blood carotenoid levels and lower numbers of cell markers of oxidative stress. Out of all the carotenoids measured, alpha-carotene, found in orange-colored vegetables, is the most predictive of lower levels of cellular oxidation, a biological precursor to many cancers.

Stone Fruits

Stone fruits include apricots, figs, peaches, plums, and nectarines. The "pits" (seeds) inside the fruit must be removed before eating.

These stone fruits contain nutrients that support breast cancer recovery.

- Apricots contain alpha-carotene, an antioxidant that can reduce precancerous cell changes which may become breast tumors.
- Apricots are also rich in lycopene, which inhibits breast cancer growth.
- Peaches contain carotenoids, and ellagic acid, which has been found to reduce the risk of estrogen-mediated breast cancer among postmenopausal women.
- Plums contain antioxidant polyphenols, shown to interfere with cancer cell replication in laboratory studies.
- Plums are currently being studied for their isatin content, which is showing promising antiproliferative effects on human breast cancer cells.

Sweeteners

Xylitol, maltitol, and erythritol are alcohol sweeteners that are non-toxic and provide health benefits. They are not only lower in carbs and contain 33 percent fewer calories than sucrose, but they also act as prebiotics by enhancing the growth of gut flora. Xylitol also reduces dental cavities by inducing remineralization of deeper layers of demineralized tooth enamel.

Carbohydrate-based sweeteners such as maple syrup, agave syrup, or brown rice syrup may be used sparingly. Avoid using refined sugar for sweetening as sugars suppress immune function and increase cancer growth.

Tea

Black, white, and green tea provide nutrients found to specifically suppress breast cancer.

Brew loose leaf or bagged tea following the package instructions: Steep the tea for just under two minutes. By removing the leaves from the brewed tea at this point, you retain the maximum amount of protective catechins without extracting undesirable components like bitter tannins and excess caffeine.

Green tea cubes can be frozen in ice cube trays to make tea cubes that can be added to smoothies. Steep green or white tea, let it cool, and then pour the tea into stainless steel or silicone ice cube trays. Once frozen, simply pop out the cubes into food storage bags where they will stay fresh in the freezer for months.

Green tea is rich in EGCG, a major green tea catechin, that suppresses breast tumor angiogenesis and growth. White tea is a rich source of catechins and polyphenols that possess strong antimutagenic properties.

Tomatoes

Whole fresh tomatoes, as well as cooked, dried, and juiced tomatoes, all provide carotenoids that help protect against breast cancer cell growth. Tomatoes contain concentrated amounts of lycopene, a carotenoid that acts as an antioxidant, reducing free radicals in the body.

Water

Proper hydration is critical to the healing process. Drink eight eight-ounce glasses of pure water each day. Tap water should be purified using a solid carbon filter or bottled filtered water in glass bottles. Avoid water provided in plastic bottles due to of the risk of phthalates.

Whole Grains

Grains are small, hard, dry seeds that are eaten cooked, and they are often ground into flour. Examples of grains include wheat, rice, quinoa, oats, kamut, teff, barley, and corn.

Whole grains supply dietary zinc, important for protection against cancer. Proper amounts of zinc are necessary for the production of enzymes that digest food. Enzymes help the body absorb nutrients and protein, promoting overall health and proper immune function. Scientists have found that higher levels of zinc from dietary sources are associated with reduced cancer risk.

Plant lignans are also found in whole grains and are associated with lowered breast cancer risk. Phytoestrogen lignans are plant compounds structurally similar to estradiol. Lignans appear to suppress the growth of breast cancer cells by reducing the tumor-stimulating effects of circulating estrogen. Studies have found that lignans are particularly effective at reducing breast cancer risk in postmenopausal women.

When shopping for grains, chose those that are whole-grain, bromine-free, and organic. Many people are sensitive to the gluten in wheat and barley. They should look for bakery products and flour that is gluten-free. Some can tolerate wheat better if it is sprouted first.

Corn

Limit corn consumption as it is contains high levels of fructose. Avoid high fructose corn syrup altogether. However, popcorn, a form of corn, is lower in sugar by weight, meaning that it takes a small number of kernels to make a serving of popcorn. Popcorn, made at home with olive oil, is a high-fiber snack food that can be enhanced nutritionally by adding nutrient-dense toppings such as spices, nutritional yeast, and garlic powder.

Oats

Plant lignans found in oats are being studied for their protective effects against breast cancer. Like other grains, oats contain lignans. Steel-cut oats are heartier than instant and carry a lower glycemic load.

Rice

Brown whole grain rice contains the phenolic compounds p-coumaric acid and protocatechuic acid and the flavonoid tricin. Eating brown rice on a regular basis may help inhibit breast cancer formation.

Warning: According to Consumer Reports, arsenic has been found in many rice products, including organic rice products. Brown rice syrup may contain high levels of arsenic while white basmati rice has the lowest levels of arsenic.

Rye

Rye provides fiber that reduces levels of toxic-free bile acids and increases the production of cancer-protective butyrate. Fiber also lowers circulating estrogens and contains bioactive compounds that are antioxidative and potentially anticarcinogenic. In addition, vitamins, minerals, and phytic acid in rye may provide protection against the development of breast cancer.

Foods to Avoid

This section covers foods and substances that should be avoided as they increase the risk for breast cancer or directly promote breast cancer cell growth.

Alcohol

Alcohol includes beer, wine, and hard liquor. Drinking alcohol increases risk for breast cancer, especially for those with estrogen-positive tumors, those who are postmenopausal, those who smoke, and those with a family history of breast cancer.

Just one alcoholic beverage per day can increase the risk for breast cancer, and heavy drinking increases risk dramatically. Women who have two to five drinks a day are at least 50 percent likelier to develop the disease.

Coffee

Coffee contains antioxidants and anticancer nutrients, however too much could be a risk. A large study of women that was conducted over twenty-two years found that drinking four cups of caffeinated coffee daily slightly increased the risk of breast cancer in postmenopausal women.

Non-organic coffee beans may contain agricultural chemicals. If you do drink coffee, make sure that it is organic.

Corn

Most varieties of corn today are genetically modified. They are high in unhealthy omega-6 fatty acids and sugars and low in nutrients. For these reasons, corn should not be a staple vegetable, but can be eaten occasionally.

Dairy

Dairy foods include cheese, yogurt, ice cream, milk, and butter. Dairy foods should be minimized as they often contain hormones from the animals themselves and possible additional hormones administered in their food and/or injected into the animals. Eating dairy foods increases serum levels of insulin-like growth factor (IGF-1). A study of over ninety thousand postmenopausal women found that higher concentrations of IGF-1 were associated with higher risk of breast cancer. Recombinant bovine somatotropin (rBST) is commonly used in dairy production and may increase risk for breast cancer by increasing IGF-1. To avoid rBST, look for organic certification, which is only given to products that do not contain rBST.

Also, organic milk from pasture-fed cows has been found to contain 25 percent less omega-6 fatty acids and 62 percent more omega-3 fatty acids. There is evidence that diets high in omega-6 and low in omega-3 increase the risk of inflammation, which may increase the risk of cancer.

If you do choose to drink or eat dairy products, be sure that they are organic, which significantly lowers the risk for those with hormone-sensitive cancer types.

Folic Acid

Studies suggest caution when taking a folic acid supplement. The Prostate, Lung, Colorectal, and Ovarian Cancer Screening Trial found a 30 percent greater breast cancer risk in women who take over 400 mcg of folic acid daily.

Folate, the naturally occurring equivalent found in many foods, was not associated with a higher risk. Folate is protective against risk for breast cancer. Higher intake of folate, B-12, and methionine slightly lowers risk for subtype ER+ breast cancer.

Avoid folic acid supplementation and increase intake of B vitamins through foods (nutritional yeast, lentils, beans, and broccoli) rather than supplements.

Meat

Those who eat red meat (beef, lamb, and pork) regularly have a higher risk of developing breast cancer. Red meat is particularly risky for adolescent girls. Those who eat red meat have a significantly higher rate of premenopausal breast cancer development, though not postmenopausal breast cancer.

The risk is not just from the foods themselves, but also from their preparation. The high heat used to fry or char meat creates heterocyclic amine compounds. These compounds are mutagenic, meaning that they activate cellular mutations and may lead to the formation and sequestering of cancer cells. Studies have linked consumption of fried meats to increased cancer incidence.

The greatest increase in risk is associated with consumption of processed meats, according to a study involving over thirty-five thousand women. Processed meats include bacon, sausage, roast beef, pepperoni, bologna, and many deli meats.

Refined Carbohydrates

Diets that limit foods made from white flour and simple sugars, as well as other processed carbohydrates, are linked to a lower likelihood of breast cancer.

Hyperglycemia occurs when there is too much circulating sugar in the bloodstream. Scientists believe that high blood glucose levels may be detrimental to the immune system and may hinder the immune-enhancing effects of the antioxidant vitamin C. Avoid refined carbohydrates, such as refined flours and simple sugars, and emphasize complex carbohydrate foods, which are high in fiber, such as vegetables, whole grains, and legumes in your diet.

Rice

Because arsenic is naturally found in soil, water, and air, it is also found in trace amounts in many fruits and vegetables. Rice is uniquely vulnerable to contamination with arsenic because it's grown in flooded fields. The rice plants soak the arsenic up through their roots and store it in the grains. To avoid ingesting too much arsenic, eat other grains. Wheat and oats have lower levels of arsenic than rice. Quinoa, millet, and amaranth are low-arsenic, gluten-free grain options.

If you do choose rice, eat it only occasionally. White basmati rice is the best option. Instant rice is also fairly low in arsenic. Arsenic levels are highest in brown rice.

Processed Foods

Foods that have been hydrogenated or contain chemicals such as food coloring, preservatives, and synthetic flavoring agents should be avoided. Opt for whole, unprocessed foods that are organic whenever possible.

Processed and high-glycemic foods that are laden with sugar should be avoided. These include candies, cakes, sweets, carbonated sodas, biscuits, ice cream, white bread, white rice, sugar, honey, marmalades, and alcohol.

Solid Fat

Fats come in many forms. Monounsaturated fats and polyunsaturated fats are the type that are liquid at room temperature and include most oils. Saturated fats are those found in animal foods such as lard and butter. Trans fats are the most unhealthy. They are primarily oils that have had hydrogen atoms added to make them solid at room temperature, for example, margarine. They are identified on food labels as "hydrogenated" or "partially hydrogenated." A diet containing high amounts of trans fats is linked to higher rates of breast cancer.

Look for monounsaturated fats for cooking such as olive oil. Research suggests that choosing monounsaturated fats may help reduce breast cancer risk in those who are postmenopausal. Avoid safflower, corn, and soy oil; all of these are high in omega-6 fatty acids.

Also, avoid processed oils, which are often oxidized by light and the heat of the processing machines. Processed oils may also contain chemicals from compounds used to extract the oils from plants and seeds. Avoid heating most oils to high temperatures as heat can cause them to form polycyclic aromatic hydrocarbons (PAHs), which are carcinogenic and very hard to break down and excrete. Also, avoid oils stored in plastic. Plastic often contains phthalates, which can leach into foods, especially fatty foods. Phthalate exposure may increase the risk of breast cancer.

Synthetic Sweeteners

Artificial or synthetic sweeteners increase glucose intolerance, and cause dysbiosis. Many are toxic and some are carcinogenic. Common chemical sweeteners include aspartame, sucralose, neotame, acesulfame potassium, saccharin, and advantame, which go by brand names such as NutraSweet, Sweet'n Low, and Splenda.

Synthetic sweeteners can trigger the liver and muscles to release stored sugar in the form of glycogen, which causes a spike in blood sugar levels. This spike may trigger the release of insulin-like growth factor, which can increase breast cancer growth.

These synthetic compounds have also been found to inhibit the growth of beneficial microbes in the intestines.

Chapter Five

MICROBIAL HEALTH

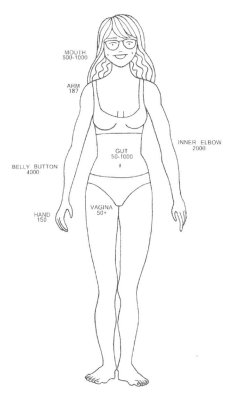

MOUTH
500-1000

ARM
187

INNER ELBOW
2000

GUT
50-1000

BELLY BUTTON
4000

HAND
150

VAGINA
50+

A staggering number of microbial species exist in and on our bodies. Scientists have only begun to identify the number of different species that colonize in specific places on the human body. The numbers above represent the average number of species known to date.

Microbes are live organisms that live in and on our bodies. Some provide essential health benefits such as supporting digestion, reducing cancer risk, affecting genetic expression, improving detoxification, reducing inflammation, and helping to minimize cancer treatment side effects. However, some organisms are pathogenic and appear to be either causative, meaning they play a role in the development of disease, or they are opportunistic, that is they have an easier time growing in a weakened system.

There is an established pattern of bacterial imbalance with human breast cancer. When we correct this imbalance by eradicating the pathogenic organisms and supplementing the normal health protective organisms, we change the internal environment and reduce the ability of cancer to grow.

Microbiota

The human microbiota refers to the collection of microbes inhabiting the human body. These organisms (mostly bacteria) live inside of us, mostly in our colon but also in smaller numbers in our small intestine and on our skin. The intestinal microbiome plays an important role in human physiology and health.

Microbiome

The human microbiome is the ecological community of symbiotic and pathogenic microorganisms that literally share our body space. These microorganisms are mostly types of bacteria, but also include fungi and other microscopic organisms. The human microbiome consists of about one hundred trillion microbial cells, outnumbering human cells ten to one. In other words, the human body contains over ten times more microbial cells than human cells. These microbes are small and although there are trillions of these organisms living in and on our bodies, their total weight is estimated to be between just one and three pounds.

Current Microbiome Research

The Human Microbiome Project (HMP) was launched in 2008 by the US National Institutes of Health with the goal of identifying and characterizing all of the human microorganisms. From this has come the collection of information we have to date on the genetic makeup of microbes that inhabit the human body. Some organisms are health supportive and necessary for our survival and some are pathogenic which means they can cause disease. Their mechanisms of action comprise a very intense area of research.

The HMP is a large-scale attempt at identifying these organisms with DNA sequencing. Although this project is ongoing, researchers have linked many pathogenic origins to specific diseases including diabetes, obesity, autism, schizophrenia, and cancer.

Future Microbiome Applications

The research being done to identify the various symbiotic, human microbes is providing the knowledge we need to be able to replace lost microbes via implants and supplementation. This research is also helping us better understand how the abnormalities in our microbial colonies lead to maldigestion, immune diseases, and malignancies.

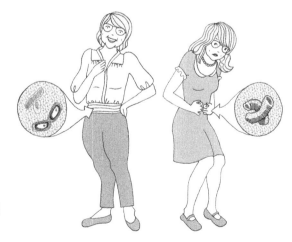

Some microbes are symbiotic and provide health benefits, while others are pathogenic and may cause illness.

Microbes and Estrogens

We need microflora to do jobs for us such as metabolizing our internally produced hormones and phytoestrogens, which are the hormones we ingest from plant foods.

Microbes and Digestion

Microbes also transform nutrients so that we can metabolize, or absorb, them properly.

Microbes and Infection

The healthful bacteria also protect us from pathogenic bacterial, fungal, and viral infections. When our healthy flora are growing and colonizing along our intestinal walls, they keep the unhealthy fungi and bacteria from adhering and growing.

They also promote immune function and, since nearly 70 percent of the immune system's function happens in the colon, these organisms can inhibit tumor formation.

Initial Colonization of Our Bodies

When we are born we have our first exposure to these healthy organisms through our mother's birth canal and through our mother's milk. As babies, we ingest more bacteria from sucking on objects, crawling on the ground, and putting our hands in our mouths. As adults we continue to colonize more bacteria in our digestive tracts by picking up organisms from foods, especially cultured or fermented foods, such as kimchi, sauerkraut, and kefir.

Antibiotics

Each organism finds a niche where it may grow for many years. When we take antibiotics, we kill off many of the bad (pathogenic) bacteria, but also the healthful organisms. Other medications also reduce the number of desired bacteria in our gut, such as NSAIDs (Non-Steroidal Anti-Inflammatory Drugs), steroids, and even chemotherapy.

Dysbiosis

Imbalance in microbial communities is called microbial dysbiosis. When the microbial ecology is disturbed from illness, medications, diet, genetic conditions, or hormonal imbalance it often leads to abnormalities.

Reduced levels of normal microbes have been found to lead to lower circulating lymphocytes and increased neutrophil-to-lymphocyte ratio, a finding which has been associated with a decreased survival in women with breast cancers.

Dysbiosis also plays a role in the recycling of estrogens via circulation through the liver, increasing the effect of estrogen, which is another leading cause of breast malignancy.

Causes of Dysbiosis

Many factors influence microbial growth. A poor diet is the leading cause of dysbiosis. Low fiber and high sugar lead to the growth of fungi and unhealthy bacteria. Also, antibiotic use greatly reduces microbial numbers of both pathogenic and healthful organisms. Stress hormones, such as cortisol, can also hinder the growth of our beneficial microbes.

Toxins such as chlorinated water damage microbes in the digestive tract. Dietary sugar feeds organisms that are harmless unless their numbers increase, at which point an overgrowth can become pathogenetic. For example, candida, proteus mirabilis, and klebsiella pneumoniae are often part of a normal healthy ecology but they all easily overgrow from exposure to dietary sugar.

Breast Protective Microbes

When researchers investigated the potential role of microbiota in breast cancer, they tested breast tumor tissue and normal tissue from the same patient. Researchers concluded that bacteria may be influencing the local immune microenvironment (Lakritz et al., 2014).

Pathogenic Bacteria and Breast Cancer

Researchers who study breast microbiota DNA found that breast cancer patients have lower numbers of helpful bacteria in their intestines and they also have a specific imbalance in the ducts in their breasts.

Microbiologists have discovered several key organisms that are in abundance in women who don't have breast cancer. This was a significant discovery and has lead researchers to test the bacteria in women who have breast cancer in the hopes that it might offer guidance in individual microorganism deficiencies. Probiotics can be supplemented and may boost protection and therapeutic benefit. Astoundingly, they have proven to offer significant protection and inhibitory effects.

They found that the bacterium *Methylobacterium radiotolerans* was common in tumor tissue, while the bacterium *Sphingomonas yanoikuyae* was common in normal healthy tissue (Caiyun et al., 2014). This is a significant finding and could lead to adjuvant treatment in which the healthy organism is replenished via supplements.

Probiotics and Breast Cancer

A recent study evaluated the immunomodulatory effects of *Lactobacillus acidophilus* (Aragón et al., 2014). Researchers found that oral administration of *Lactobacillus* provided antitumor support as it reduced tumor growth rate and increased lymphocyte proliferation.

The Standard American Diet (SAD) does not support healthy microbial gut growth. SAD is low in fruits, vegetables, legumes, and whole grains, and high in processed foods, sugar, and artificial sweeteners.

Cultured foods contain naturally occurring bacteria, such as those found in sourdough, and those with culture added, such as cultured coconut milk, cultured, kimchi, tempeh, and miso.

Probiotics Defined

Probiotics are beneficial bacteria (sometimes referred to as "friendly germs") that help to maintain the health of the intestinal tract and aid in digestion. They also help keep potentially harmful bacteria and yeasts under control. Most probiotics come from food sources, especially cultured milk products. Probiotics can be taken as capsules, tablets, and powders, or consumed in cultured foods and beverages.

Prebiotics Defined

Probiotics should not be confused with prebiotics. Prebiotics are complex sugars (such as lactulose, lactitol, a variety of fructo-oligosaccharides, and inulin) that are used as fuel by healthful bacteria to stimulate their growth and activity while suppressing the growth and activity of harmful organisms. Other foods that may support probiotic activity include Japanese miso, tempeh, kefir, raw milk, kombucha, bananas, garlic, and onions. When prebiotics and probiotics are combined in one product, it is called a synbiotic.

Non-digestible carbohydrates act as prebiotics that stimulate the growth of certain intestinal bacteria that support healthy colon conditions. A couple of effective prebiotics are fructooligosaccharides and digestive-resistant maltodextrin that were found to inhibit tumor growth and spread. Prebiotics have also been found to increase apoptosis. These probiotics also provide an epigenetic effect on tumor expression genes. They have been found to have a particularly protective effect against ER+ tumors.

Probiotics are thought to work by colonizing the small intestine and crowding out disease-causing organisms, thereby restoring proper balance to the intestinal flora. They compete with unhealthy organisms for nutrients and may also produce substances that inhibit growth of pathogenic organisms in the gut.

Probiotic bacteria have been found to stimulate the body's immune system. They may also aid in several gastrointestinal illnesses such as inflammatory bowel diseases, antibiotic-related diarrhea, *Clostridium difficile* toxin-induced colitis, infectious diarrhea, hepatic encephalopathy, irritable bowel syndrome, and allergies.

Internal Ecology and Digestion

Probiotics have been found to enhance the digestion and absorption of proteins, fats, calcium, and phosphorus. They may also help overcome lactose intolerance and restore healthful bacteria after a course of antibiotic therapy has altered the normal gastrointestinal flora.

Lactobacillus casei

An exciting breast cancer study found that the probiotic supplement *Lactobacillus casei* was found to delay or block tumor development via modulation of the immune response.

Lactobacillus acidophilus

Lactobacilli are a normal part of the flora in a healthy colon. They have been found to boost immune function and protect against malignancies. The immunomodulatory effects of *Lactobacillus acidophilus* alters the cytokine production, enhancing antitumor immunity by reducing the tumor growth rate and increasing lymphocyte proliferation.

Sources: Supplements, some probiotic cultured products

Lactobacillus reuteri

Lactobacillus reuteri is an important bacterial organism in breast tissue which has been found to provide protection against cancer development as well as significantly inhibit the growth of existing breast cancer.

This probiotic protects against the progression of breast cancer. Some nutrients become genetic triggers when activated by microbes. For example, anthocyanins from fruits and vegetables become bioactive when they are metabolized by bacteria in the gut. These activated anthocyanins have the ability to turn on tumor suppressor genes.

This discovery is so compelling that researchers are considering the use of *L. reuteri* supplementation, an effective public health approach to help counteract the accumulated dietary and genetic carcinogenic events integral in the Westernized diet and lifestyle.

Lactobacillus plantarum

Supplements that contain *Lactobacillus plantarum* provide protection against breast cancer development. *Lactobacillus* may be even more effective when combined with inulin, a prebiotic that supports the growth of probiotics.

Our Own Personal Microbiome

Laboratory tests such as a microbiology stool assessment analyze an individuals healthy as well as pathogenic organisms (bacteria, fungi, and parasites). The lab test results include a report that not only identifies which pathogenic organisms you have, but also provides a list of possible treatments for eradicating them.

▌ STRATEGY: MICROBIAL HEALTH CHAPTER

Increase fermented foods in your diet and be aware that factors such as medication stress and cancer treatments can reduce the healthy levels of your gut flora.

CHECKLIST

- Order a Microbiology Analysis kit (bacterial and fungal test). If your doctor does not currently offer these, visit my website daniellachace.com for order information.
- Once you receive your test results, follow the recommendations for both eradicating pathogenic organisms and supplementing with probiotics.

For more support in locating a physician, finding these tests, and keeping informed about microbes involved in breast cancer, visit www.daniellachace.com.

Chapter Six

SUPPLEMENTS

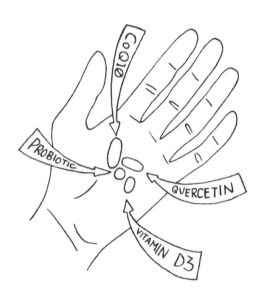

RECOMMENDED SUPPLEMENTS

Coenzyme Q10	Probiotics
Creatine	Quercetin
Iodine	Riboflavin
Licorice	Selenium
Modified Citrus Pectin	Vitamin C
Melatonin	Vitamin D3
NAC	Zinc

A whole foods, plant-based diet supplies most of the nutrients needed on a daily basis. However, there are specific situations when food does not provide enough of the nutrients we need and deficiencies develop. We have an increased need for nutrients during illness, treatment, and healing periods. Many medications also deplete nutrients, which may lead to deficiencies.

Physical symptoms give us initial clues about nutrient deficiencies, but lab tests are needed to positively identify vitamin and mineral levels. Those at varying stages of breast cancer, whether working toward healing or preventing reoccurrence, should be tested for deficiencies and then supplemented to meet the needs identified by the lab tests.

Oral supplements are widely available, and high-quality, absorbable nutrients are effective at boosting nutrient levels quickly. The source, form, and dosage are all are all important in choosing nutrients that will ultimately be bioactive and effective.

Probiotic supplements are also frequently needed until the organisms adhere in the colon and grow to sufficient levels. Once they have colonized, they will continue to grow on their own, and supplementation is no longer necessary. These gastrointestinal organisms are needed for proper epigenetic activity.

A microbiology stool test provides accurate identification of the organisms currently in an individual's colon. This stool test provides information about the levels of healthful organisms and those that may be pathogenic. Many laboratories provide sensitivity testing to determine the most effective treatment for the pathogenic organisms. Lab results now include the new information coming from the National Institutes of Health (NIH) Human Microbiome Project (HMP). Optimizing the internal ecology enhances digestion, nutrient absorption, detoxification, and genetic methylation.

Each of the nutrients listed below support specific actions against breast cancer. Vitamin D and iodine are critical for prevention of breast cancer as well as healing. The most effective way to determine your personal needs is through nutrient deficiency blood tests.

Short of this, low dose supplementation provides a constant intake to reduce risk of deficiency.

Breast cancer patients have a greater need for certain nutrients than the general population. The doses recommended below are based on breast cancer studies. Nutrient supplements that have an adverse effect on breast cancer are listed with explanations for why they should be avoided.

Coenzyme Q10

Coenzyme Q10 (CoQ10) is a fat-soluble antioxidant that provides protection against development of breast cancer. Researchers have found that women who have low levels of CoQ10 in their blood have a higher risk for developing breast cancer.

Levels of CoQ10 drop as we age and can be depleted by medications such as statin drugs. Low levels of CoQ10 are associated with increased cancer incidence and poor recovery (Cooney et al., 2011). Coenzyme Q10 is critical to production of adenosine triphosphate (ATP) and energy production (Lance et al., 2012). CoQ10 levels can be increased with supplementation, which is effective in treating oxidative stress in those who have low circulating levels in their blood.

CoQ10 supplementation also provides therapeutic actions for breast cancer treatment as it has been found to program cancer cells to self-destruct via apoptosis.

CoQ10 supplementation appears to enhance tamoxifen therapy by restoring mitochondrial function and reducing tumor necrosis factor. A supplement containing coenzyme Q10, riboflavin, and niacin was found to reduce markers of breast cancer cells in those also taking tamoxifen (Premkumar et al., 2007; Yuvaraj et al., 2008).

CoQ10 is an important antioxidant that provides tremendous protective benefits with no known risk, and warrants addition to breast cancer prevention and/or treatment plans.

Recommendation: 100 mg per day

Creatine

Creatine and branched-chain amino acids (BCAAs) can significantly enhance muscle development (de Campos-Ferraz et al., 2014). Daily supplementation with creatine powders reduces muscle loss and has proven effective in cachexia prevention and treatment.

Recommendation: 500 grams

Modified Citrus Pectin

Modified citrus pectin (MCP), is a nondigestible, water-soluble polysaccharide fiber derived from citrus fruit found to inhibit breast tumor growth and metastasis (Nangia-Makker et al., 2002). Modified citrus pectin (MCP) is also known as fractionated citrus pectin, and fractionated pectin powder and sometimes just fractionated pectin. It is a complex polysaccharide obtained from the peel and pulp of citrus fruits. MCP is rich in galactoside residues. Metastasis is one of the most life-threatening aspects of cancer and the lack of effective anti-metastatic therapies has prompted research on MCP's effectiveness in blocking metastasis of certain types of cancers, including melanomas, prostate, and breast.

MCP's apparent safety and proven anti-metastatic action, and the lack of other proven therapies against metastasis, justifies its inclusion in comprehensive orthomolecular anticancer regimens.

These galactoside residues can preferentially bind to the lectins on the cell membranes of the unwanted cells, in turn preventing the attachment of the unwanted cells to normal cells, thus inhibiting the growth of these cells.

Recommendation: 5 grams, twice per day

Iodine

Iodine is an antioxidant and antiproliferative agent contributing to the integrity of normal mammary glands. All breast cancer patients should be tested for iodine deficiency and supplemented with iodine as needed.

Supplementation exerts a suppressive effect on the growth and size of both benign and cancerous growths.

Iodine deficiency can lead to hypothyroidism, which can cause fatigue, low body temperature, foggy brain, increase in body fat, brittle hair, and lowered immune function.

If you suspect you may have an iodine deficiency, ask your doctor for a blood test to confirm. Boost iodine in your diet with iodized salt and consider taking an iodine supplement.

Many practitioners are finding high doses of iodine effective in reversal of hyperthyroidism. If you learn that you have low thyroid from lab tests, seek the advice of your oncologist or an integrative medical professional to help you determine the right therapeutic dose.

Recommendation: 225 mcg per day

Licorice

Endocrine-disrupting chemicals (EDCs) have been reported to interfere with estrogen signaling. Exposure to these chemicals decreases the immune response and causes a wide range of diseases in animals and humans. Many studies have shown that licorice root (*Glycyrrhiza glabra*) extract exhibits antioxidative, chemoprotective, and detoxifying properties.

Licorice root extract can be used as a potential toxicity-alleviating agent against endocrine-disrupting chemicals (Chu et al., 2014). Licorice, however, can raise blood pressure levels in those with pre-existing hypertension. Therefore, those with high blood pressure should use a modified licorice product called deglycerized licorice.

Melatonin

Early studies indicate that melatonin supplementation may be useful for breast cancer prevention and treatment by reducing breast cancer cell growth. Melatonin supplementation has been found to reduce breast cancer cell growth and increases cancer cell destruction by modulating estrogen-dependent pathways that lead to cancer cell growth.

Artificial light at night (ALAN) leads to melatonin suppression and deficiency. Low levels of melatonin effect methylation of genes and has been found to cause epigenetic triggering involved in breast cancer (Haim et al., 2015). Researchers are quick to point out that this ALAN-induced epigenetic modification is reversible, therefore early detection is of great significance in the treatment of breast cancer. Melatonin levels can be monitored with saliva and blood tests.

Those who are deficient can be treated with melatonin supplementation. Once normal levels of melatonin have been restored, supplements are no longer necessary. Levels can be maintained with proper sleep and a melatonin-rich diet. Melatonin not only acts as an antioxidant, blocks estrogen receptors, and triggers apoptosis, but also reverses epigenetic triggers, thus turning off breast cancer pathways.

Melatonin supplementation has proven to improve survival rate and toleration of treatment, especially for those who are ER+ (Martinez-Campa et al., 2008).

Recommendation: 20 mg of melatonin at bedtime

N-acetyl Cysteine

N-acetyl cysteine (NAC) is an important sulfur-containing amino acid utilized in many metabolic pathways. Cysteine is a powerful antioxidant and detoxifier as a precursor (a substance that precedes another) for glutathione enzymes, which the body, especially the liver, uses for disabling destructive free radicals.

NAC provides protection from chemical toxicity and supports the detoxification process in smokers and people exposed to chemicals or air pollution.

Cysteine is found in oats, and wheat germ, and in sulfur-containing foods such as garlic, onions, and broccoli.

Recommendation: 250 mg, twice per day

Probiotics

Hundreds of different strains of beneficial microorganisms live in our digestive tract. Many have been found to provide direct benefit in protection against breast cancer. For example, *Lactobacillus acidophilus* has a suppressive effect on tumors by stimulating the production of immunologic factors.

Suggested strains: *Bifidobacterium breve, Bifidobacterium longum, Bifidobacterium infantis, Lactobacillus acidophilus, Lactobacillus plantarum, Lactobacillus paracasei, Lactobacillus bulgaricus,* and *Streptococcus thermophilus.*

Sacro-B *(Saccharomyces boulardii)* is a particularly hearty strain that can be taken during chemotherapy, radiation, and while taking pharmaceutical medications. Sacro-B supplementation is also an effective treatment for *Clostridium difficile.* Many other strains are more delicate and may be damaged or killed by treatments and medications. Sacro-B can act as a placeholder when other strains would not survive in the body. Some treatments and medications reduce the numbers of these healthy organisms. After treatments and medications are completed, a high dose, broad range probiotic supplement can replace the Sacro-B.

Probiotic supplement brands that adhere in the gut and, therefore, benefit provide the most benefit are Thorne Research, Klaire Labs, and Integrative Therapeutics. There are others, but these are the products that I have used clinically over the last twenty years and have confirmed their colonization via stool tests. Unfortunately, many probiotic products do not colonize well, so I use the few that have proven to be live, active cultures.

Recommendation: Probiotic (20 billion+ in each capsule), twice per day

Recommendation: *Saccharomyces boulardii,* 250 mg per day

Quercetin

Quercetin is a polyphenolic bioflavonoid that inhibits cell growth and induces apoptosis in lab tests on human breast cancer cells and inhibits development of both primary and recurrent breast cancer. Quercetin also suppresses angiogenesis and supports immune function. Quercetin has also been found to have an epigenetic effect in turning off angiogenesis pathways (Xioa et al., 2011).

Quercetin is recommended for supporting BPA (Bisphenol A) detoxification. BPA is a potential breast cancer initiator, therefore it is a high-risk toxin. Quercetin supports clearance of BPA from our blood and body tissues and is an effective detoxifier of BPA. Most of us have been exposed to this toxin throughout our lives.

Recommendation: 500 mg per day

Riboflavin

Riboflavin supplementation taken in conjunction with tamoxifen treatment can help reduce damage to the liver that can occur as a side effect. Tamoxifen, a drug used to treat breast cancer, can cause liver damage in some people. Women who took a supplement containing riboflavin for ninety days as an adjunct to tamoxifen had reduced markers of cellular oxidative stress, reflecting a protective effect of riboflavin on liver health. Riboflavin, also known as B2, is commonly found in many multivitamin supplements. It works synergistically with other B vitamins and should be taken as part of a B complex.

Recommendation: 10 mg per day

Selenium

Selenium plays an important role in detoxification and may help prevent breast cancer. Toxic elements in the environment can accumulate in the body and may contribute to the proliferation of cancerous cells. Selenium plays an important role in detoxifying the body by keeping the concentration of elements at safe levels.

Recommendation: 200 mcg per day

Vitamin C

Hyperglycemia (high blood sugar) has been linked to vitamin C deficiency, which can impair immune function in patients with cancer. Maintaining optimal levels of ascorbic acid (vitamin C) is important for immune function. Higher levels of blood glucose appears to decrease cellular stores of ascorbic acid. Impaired immune function is often the result. Reduce sugar intake, as hyperglycemia is common in cancer patients, and increase vitamin C–rich foods and supplement with vitamin C to ensure adequate intake throughout treatment.

Recommendation: 1 gram, twice per day

Vitamin D3

D3 is a hormone and needed for immune function. All breast cancer patients should be tested for vitamin D deficiency and supplement with vitamin D3 as needed. Breast cancer risk was found to be 45 percent lower in women with high vitamin D blood concentrations. Vitamin D acts as a cancer protective agent by exerting anti-proliferative effects on cancerous cells.

Vitamin D affects breast cancer to a degree that it is being described as a "vitamin D deficiency syndrome." Researchers have discovered that those with the lowest vitamin D levels are at the highest risk, while those with the highest vitamin D levels have the highest survival rate and the least reoccurrence, and studies have shown a 66 percent lower risk of metastasis with normal D level.

Once your vitamin D is up to a healthy level, reduce your intake to a maintenance dose with either a 2000 IU (Vitamin D3 cholecalciferol) daily supplement or with a vitamin D promoting lifestyle, which includes 15 minutes of direct sun on your skin each day and foods rich in D, such as fortified -orange juice, -rice milk, -soy milk, or -almond milk and mushrooms.

Vitamin D affects the structure of cells involved in breast cancer. It holds certain breast cells together with a glue-like substance called E-cadherin, which provides structure to the cell. E-cadherin is made up of mostly vitamin D and calcium. Replenishing vitamin D supports breast cell structure and improves immune function, which can substantially reduce breast cancer cell growth.

Recent studies suggest adults need about 8,000 IU of vitamin D3 per day in order to get serum levels above 40 ng/mL. A blood test is necessary to determine your circulating blood levels. Be sure to request that your medical provider perform this test if you have not had a vitamin D test within the last year.

Blood levels: Goal 50 to 70 ng/mL

Recommendation: 2,000 IU of vitamin D3 per day for maintenance. Higher levels of supplementation are needed to reverse a deficiency.

Food Sources of Zinc

SERVING SIZE	FOOD	ZINC (mg)
3 ounces	Pumpkin seeds	8
3 ounces	Cashews	5
3 ounces	Popcorn	4
3 ounces	Peanuts	3
6 ounces	Baked beans	3

Zinc

Zinc is a mineral necessary for immune function, cell development, wound repair, enzyme production, the formation of insulin, and carbohydrate digestion. Maintaining healthy zinc levels also provides protection from the effects of estrogen on breast cancer cells.

Symptoms of zinc deficiency include low energy, suppressed immune function, acne, eczema, loss of taste, high cholesterol levels, prolonged wound healing, brittle nails/white spots on nails, hair loss, skin problems, poor digestion, GERD (gastric esophageal reflux disease), and fatigue.

Zinc is provided in many multivitamin/mineral products. The most easily assimilated form is zinc picolinate.

Recommendation: 15 mg per day

▌STRATEGY: SUPPLEMENT CHAPTER

Ensure that you are not currently deficient in any of the key nutrients needed for healing by seeking advice from a professional, testing, supplementing to reverse deficiencies as needed and by eating a nutrient rich diet to reduce the chances of developing a deficiency in the future.

CHECKLIST

- Consider meeting with a naturopathic doctor (ND) or nutritionist to review your current supplement program and to discuss whether you would benefit from nutrient supplementation, such as vitamins, minerals and amino acids. This will most likely be determined by identifying nutrient deficiencies with blood tests.
- Everyone living in North America who is at risk for, or has been diagnosed with, breast cancer should know whether they need to be supplementing with vitamin D3. Most doctors routinely check for vitamin D deficiency these days, but it is important that you ask your doctor if you have been tested. If you haven't been tested in the last year, ask your doctor for this test.
- If you take other medications or are experiencing side effects of treatment, an ND or nutritionist can help you determine

nutrients that are likely to be needed, even without blood tests. For example, if you take a medication known to deplete nutrients such as statin drugs, which deplete CoQ10, your clinician may recommend that you start taking that nutrient without confirming a deficiency with lab tests.

- Also if you are experiencing deficiency symptoms such as cachexia, your clinician may recommend that you take creatine for several weeks prior to testing. This way the blood or urine test is used to confirm that the protein supplement has increased your amino acid uptake and muscle development.

- Some supplements are safe and gentle and can be taken without testing, such as modified citrus pectin, deglycerized licorice, probiotics, and quercetin. These are safe to take without consulting an expert and can be purchased from most grocery stores, pharmacies and from many clinics.

- If you are not sleeping well, take measures to improve sleep and consider a saliva test for melatonin levels.

For more support in locating a physician, finding these tests, and keeping informed about supplement recommendations, visit www.daniellachace.com.

Chapter Seven

SELF-CARE

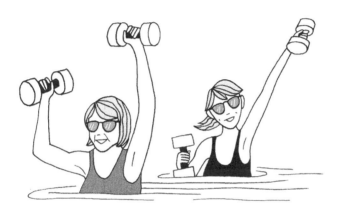

Self-care includes a consistent practice of exercise, maintaining a healthy weight, stress reduction, adequate sleep, and socializing, along with physical and emotional therapies like meditation, music, yoga, and massage. These are proven therapies that improve outcome.

Exercise

Exercise supports detoxification and boosts immune function, enhancing metabolism, strengthening our muscles, and improving oxygenation of our tissues.

Exercise not only reduces body fat but also reduces insulin resistance, which is a risk factor in the development of breast cancer.

Insulin resistance also exacerbates existing cancer development (Ghose et al., 2015).

Women who exercise vigorously for seven or more hours each week have a 25 percent drop in breast cancer risk, compared to those who exercise less than one hour each week. Examples of vigorous activity include basketball, swimming, and running. The results were similar if women walked briskly, but there was no benefit for walking at a normal pace.

Exercise helps those with TNBC by improving quality of life and physical function as well as reducing body fat (Swisher et al., 2015).

Studies have shown that a 30-minute brisk walk daily reduces breast cancer mortality risk by half over a ten-year period.

Recommendation: 30-minute brisk walk daily

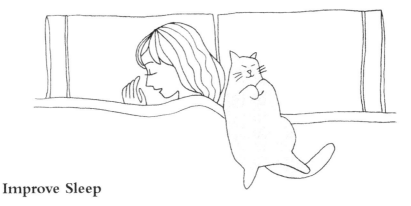

Improve Sleep

Adequate and quality sleep are critical to the healing process. Inadequate and inconsistent sleep cause circadian disruption, which is associated with an increased breast cancer risk (Rabstein et al., 2014).

Lack of sleep over time (less than six hours a night) has been noted to increase the risk of breast cancer by 62 percent. Sleep is important in regulating melatonin, an antioxidant that provides protection from breast cancer (Malina et al., 2013). When we sleep deeply, our endocrine system can recharge, which involves the nocturnal pineal production of melatonin.

Sleep with the natural light, which means getting to bed early in a dark, cool, and quiet space. Make sure to block the outside light and see that there are no lights visible, even small ones such as tiny lights on a TV or an alarm clock. Researchers found that even dim light at night interrupts circadian cycles and suppresses melatonin.

Suppressed melatonin can lead to hyperglycemia (high blood sugar), hyperinsulinemia, lipid signaling, and proliferative activity in tumors (Blask et al., 2014). A disruption in circadian sleep cycles alters core body temperature, hormone regulation, and patterns of gene expression throughout the body (Stevens et al., 2015).

Melatonin and Tamoxifen

Exposure to light at night, which shuts off nighttime production of the hormone melatonin, renders breast cancer resistant to tamoxifen, a widely used breast cancer drug. Researchers report that melatonin by itself delayed the formation of tumors and significantly slowed their growth. They also found that tamoxifen was enhanced by sleep and supplementation. Nighttime levels of melatonin boosted by complete darkness and also animal subjects receiving melatonin supplementation, even during exposure to dim light at night experienced a reduction in tumors (Dauchy et al., 2014).

Massage

Massage and touch therapies improve relaxation and comfort and support stress reduction. Lymphatic massage may also be recommended after surgery for improving circulation, lymphedema-related swelling, and discomfort (Leung et al., 2015). Overall gentle effleurage helps reduce tension and improve circulation.

Meditation

Practicing mindful meditation or being involved in a support group has a positive physical impact at the cellular level in breast cancer survivors.

Integrative mindfulness therapies have been found to improve physical and emotional health as well as social functioning after treatment. Not only does meditation improve functioning but it also helps reduce cancer-related symptoms including fatigue, pain, insomnia, constipation, anxiety, and depression (Dobos et al., 2015).

Optimal Weight

Body weight plays a significant role in breast cancer risk as obesity is responsible for one in five diagnoses of breast cancer and one in six deaths. Obesity promotes existing tumor growth by increasing inflammation and insulin resistance. Body fat also increases breast cancer development by increasing production of estrogen (Vicennati et al., 2015).

Overweight and obesity are associated with an increased risk of postmenopausal breast cancer and less favorable prognosis after diagnosis and initial treatment. Diet, toxins, and microbes all play a role in obesity. Interventions as previously discussed, such as dietary changes, detoxification, and microbial supplementation, along with exercise, can help maintain a healthy body weight and reduce risk of development as well as recurrence of breast cancer.

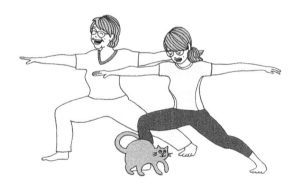

Stress Reduction

High stress events, chronic stress, depression, and poor social support increase risk for breast cancer by ninefold. Anxiety increases stress hormones such as cortisol and depletes antioxidants. This elevated state of chronic stress is now considered a carcinogenic state. Stress also alters BRCA gene expression.

Stress is inherently part of the process of hearing the diagnosis, entering the medical system, dealing with ongoing medical visits and expenses, and all of the other changes needed to navigate disease. However, it is possible to manage stress even in the face of all this.

Effective stress-reducing techniques include yoga, exercise, meditation, breathing work, and massage.

I have also learned from my clients how important boundary setting is for creating the buffer zone of protection from outside influences, time demands, and expectations. A health crisis inherently involves family, friends, a medical team, and the help of others. So there is a tremendous amount of communication happening during the process. Non-violent communication (NVC) is a system for communicating clearly and getting your needs met. It is worth learning NVC language as it is important that you are being heard and having your needs met during the healing process. Many of my clients have found that through NVC language they are able to express their needs, get the help they want, and create a buffer zone of protection from unnecessary conflict. They also report that they recognize imbalances in personal relationships sooner so they can be addressed before they cause problems.

■ STRATEGY: SELF-CARE CHAPTER

Incorporate as many of the lifestyle changes as you can comfortably manage as they each add to your quality of life and improve the recovery process, giving you more energy and reducing fatigue. These strategies will also improve the effectiveness of treatment and overall outcome.

CHECKLIST

- Choose an exercise program you enjoy and make it part of every day.
- Create a restful sleep environment (dark and comfortable).
- Try guided meditation or join a mediation group until you learn a basic thirty-minute daily practice.
- Talk to your doctor or nutritionist to determine your optimal weight and develop a weight loss plan if needed.
- Learn the basic tenets of NVC if you need help with setting boundaries.

For more support in locating practitioners, finding self-care resources, and to keeping informed about integrative care, visit www. daniellachace.com.

Physiology in Flux

We have many systems in place in our complex human bodies that repair and rebalance to bring us back to a healthy and thriving state of being. Our cells are turning over constantly, as old and damaged cells die and new healthy cells form and take their place. Keep in mind that we are healing every moment.

Effective Strategies

Breast cancer is the result of a state of imbalance. By exploring your underlying personal imbalances and taking steps to correct them, you can re-balance your body and turn off many of the genetic pathways that lead to breast cancer.

Healing Journey

My clients often report an increase in energy and quicker healing time as they remove toxins and boost nutrients in their bodies. We each seem to find the steps that make the most profound difference in our own recovery. Sharing these stories can help others to feel hopeful, even when they are just beginning the process. If you would like to send me a brief note about your healing journey, I would love to share it with others to inspire and encourage them along the path.

New Research

There is a tremendous amount of ongoing research being published about microbes, toxins, nutrients, and epigenetics in relation to breast cancer. I will continue to summarize the vast amount of information for you and will translate it into actions that you can take to apply it in your life. I will be posting recipes, nutrient studies, links to new lab tests and to clinics that offer the tests recommended throughout the book on my website, www.daniellachace.com.

REFERENCES

The references to the original work that informed the recommendations made throughout the book are provided below so that you and your medical team can access the abstracts and original research yourselves on www. PubMed.gov, which is the United States National Library of Medicine and the National Institute of Health's website.

Chapter Two: GENETICS

Baek SH, Kim SM, Nam D, Lee JH, Ahn KS, Choi SH, Kim SH, Shim BS, Chang IM, Ahn KS. (2012) Antimetastatic effect of nobiletin through the down-regulation of CXC chemokine receptor type 4 and matrix metallopeptidase-9. *Pharmaceutical Biology*.

Bailey ST, Shin H, Westerling T, Liu XS, Brown M. (2012) Estrogen receptor prevents p53-dependent apoptosis in breast cancer. *Proceedings of the National Academy of Sciences USA*.

Balleine RL, Wilcken NR. (2012) High-risk estrogen-receptor-positive breast cancer: identification and implications for therapy. *Molecular Diagnosis and Therapy*.

Basse C, Arock M. (2014) The increasing roles of epigenetics in breast cancer: Implications for pathogenicity, biomarkers, prevention and treatment. *International Journal of Cancer*.

Choi SW, Friso S. (2010) Epigenetics: A New Bridge between Nutrition and Health. *Advances in Nutrition*

Cox DG, et al. (2011) Common variants of the BRCA1 wild-type allele modify the risk of breast cancer in BRCA1 mutation carriers. *Human Molecular Genetics.*

Crujeiras AB, Díaz-Lagares A, Carreira MC, Amil M, Casanueva FF. (2013) Oxidative stress associated to dysfunctional adipose tissue: a potential link between obesity, type 2 diabetes mellitus and breast cancer. *Free Radical Research.*

Dagdemir A, Durif J, Ngollo M, Bignon YJ, Bernard-Gallon D. (2013) Histone lysine trimethylation or acetylation can be modulated by phytoestrogen, estrogen or anti-HDAC in breast cancer cell lines. *Epigenomics.*

Day TK, Bianco-Miotto T. (2013) Common gene pathways and families altered by DNA methylation in breast and prostate cancers. *Endocrine-Related Cancer.*

Deb G, Thakur VS, Gupta S. (2013) Multifaceted role of EZH2 in breast and prostate tumorigenesis: Epigenetics and beyond. *Epigenetics.*

Dumitrescu RG. (2012) Epigenetic markers of early tumor development. *Methods in Molecular Biology.*

Einbond LS, Wu HA, Kashiwazaki R, He K, Roller M, Su T, Wang X, Goldsberry S. (2012) Carnosic acid inhibits the growth of ER-negative human breast cancer cells and synergizes with curcumin. *Fitoterapia.*

Fernandez SV, Huang Y, Snider KE, Zhou Y, Pogash TJ, Russo J. (2012) Expression and DNA methylation changes in human breast epithelial cells after bisphenol A exposure. *International Journal of Oncology.*

Hartmaier RJ, Priedigkeit N, Lee AV. (2012) Who's driving anyway? Herculean efforts to identify the drivers of breast cancer. *Breast Cancer Research.*

Hervouet E, Cartron PF, Jouvenot M, Delage-Mourroux R. (2013) Epigenetic regulation of estrogen signaling in breast cancer. *Epigenetics.*

Heyn H, Carmona FJ, Gomez A, Ferreira HJ, Bell JT, Sayols S, Ward K, Stefansson OA, Moran S, Sandoval J, Eyfjord JE, Spector TD, Esteller M. (2013) DNA methylation profiling in breast cancer discordant identical twins identifies DOK7 as novel epigenetic biomarker. *Carcinogenesis.*

Veeck J, Esteller M. (2010) Breast Cancer Epigenetics: From DNA Methylation to microRNAs. *Journal of Mammary Gland Biology and Neoplasia.*

Kanaya N, Adams L, Takasaki A, Chen S. (2014) Whole blueberry powder inhibits metastasis of triple negative breast cancer in a xenograft mouse model through modulation of inflammatory cytokines. *Nutrition and Cancer.*

Kemp, Christopher J., et al. (2014) CTCF Haploinsufficiency Destabilizes DNA Methylation and Predisposes to Cancer. *Cell Reports.*

Knower KC, To SQ, Clyne CD. (2013) Intracrine oestrogen production and action in breast cancer: An epigenetic focus. *Journal of Steroid Biochemistry and Molecular Biology.*

Kwan ML. (2008) Dietary patterns and breast cancer recurrence and survival among women with early-stage breast cancer. *Journal of Clinical Oncology.*

Lee SA, et al. (2008) Cruciferous vegetables, the GSTP1 Ile105Val genetic polymorphism, and breast cancer risk. *American Journal of Clinical Nutrition.*

Li H, Yang B, Huang J, Xiang T, Yin X, Wan J, Luo F, Zhang L, Li H, Ren G. (2013) Naringin inhibits growth potential of human triple-negative breast cancer cells by targeting β–catenin signaling pathway. *Toxicology Letters.*

Luo J, Gao YT, Chow WH, Shu XO, Li H, Yang G, Cai Q, Li G, Rothman N, Cai H, Shrubsole MJ, Franke AA, Zheng W, Dai Q. (2012) Urinary polyphenols, glutathione S-transferases copy number variation, and breast cancer risk: results from the Shanghai women's health study. *Molecular Carcinogenesis.*

Miller JA, Lang JE, Ley M, Nagle R, Hsu CH, Thompson PA, Cordova C, Waer A, Chow HH. (2013) Human breast tissue disposition and bioactivity of limonene in women with early-stage breast cancer. *Cancer Prevention Research (Philadelphia).*

Mo Q, Wang S, Seshan VE, Olshen AB, Schultz N, Sander C, Powers RS, Ladanyi M, Shen R. (2013) Pattern discovery and cancer gene identification in integrated cancer genomic data. *Proceedings of the National Academy of Sciences USA.*

Ogino S, Lochhead P, Chan AT, Nishihara R, Cho E, Wolpin BM, Meyerhardt JA, Meissner A, Schernhammer ES, Fuchs CS, Giovannucci E. (2013) Molecular pathological epidemiology of epigenetics: emerging integrative science to analyze environment, host, and disease. *Modern Pathology.*

Park CJ, Nah WH, Lee JE, Oh YS, Gye MC. (2012) Butyl paraben-induced changes in DNA methylation in rat epididymal spermatozoa. *Andrologia.*

Pogash TJ, El-Bayoumy K, Amin S, Gowda K, de Cicco RL, Barton M, Su Y, Russo IH, Himmelberger JA, Slifker M, Manni A, Russo J. (2015) Oxidized derivative of docosahexaenoic acid preferentially inhibit cell proliferation in triple negative over luminal breast cancer cells. *In Vitro Cellular & Developmental Biology - Animal.*

Sieri S, et al. (2014) Dietary Fat Intake and Development of Specific Breast Cancer Subtypes. *Journal of the National Cancer Institute.*

Singh S, Li SS. (2012) Epigenetic effects of environmental chemicals bisphenol a and phthalates. *International Journal of Molecular Sciences.*

Stefansson OA, Villanueva A, Vidal A, Martí L, Esteller M. (2012) BRCA1 epigenetic inactivation predicts sensitivity to platinum-based chemotherapy in breast and ovarian cancer. *Epigenetics.*

Teegarden D, Romieu I, Lelièvre SA. (2012) Redefining the impact of nutrition on breast cancer incidence: is epigenetics involved? *Nutrition Research Reviews.*

Zhang L, Yang M, Gan L, He T, Xiao X, Stewart MD, Liu X, Yang L, Zhang T, Zhao Y, Fu J. (2012) DLX4 Upregulates TWIST and Enhances Tumor Migration, Invasion and Metastasis. *International Journal of Biological Sciences.*

Chapter Three: DETOXIFY

Abdull Razis AF, Noor NM. (2013) Cruciferous vegetables: dietary phytochemicals for cancer prevention. *Asian Pacific Journal of Cancer Prevention.*

Aceves C, Anguiano B, Delgado G. (2005) Is iodine a gatekeeper of the integrity of the mammary gland? *Journal of Mammary Gland Biology and Neoplasia.*

Alatise OI, Schrauzer GN. (2010) Lead exposure: a contributing cause of the current breast cancer epidemic in Nigerian women. *Biological Trace Element Research.*

Andra SS, Charisiadis P, Makris KC. (2014) Obesity-mediated association between exposure to brominated trihalomethanes and type II diabetes mellitus: an exploratory analysis. *Science of the Total Environment.*

Aquino NB, Sevigny MB, Sabangan J, Louie MC. (2012) The role of cadmium and nickel in estrogen receptor signaling and breast cancer: metalloestrogens or not? *Journal of Environmental Science and Health Part C Environmental Carcinogenesis & Ecotoxicology Reviews.*

Baek SH, Kim SM, Nam D, Lee JH, Ahn KS, Choi SH, Kim SH, Shim BS, Chang IM, Ahn KS. (2012) Antimetastatic effect of nobiletin through the down-regulation of CXC chemokine receptor type 4 and matrix metallopeptidase-9. *Pharmaceutical Biology.*

Betancourt AM, Wang J, Jenkins S, Mobley J, Russo J, Lamartiniere CA. (2012) Altered carcinogenesis and proteome in mammary glands of rats after prepubertal exposures to the hormonally active chemicals bisphenol a and genistein. *Journal of Nutrition.*

Bidgoli SA, Eftekhari T, Sadeghipour R. (2011) Role of xenoestrogens and endogenous sources of estrogens on the occurrence of premenopausal breast cancer in Iran. *Asian Pacific Journal of Cancer Prevention.*

Błędzka D, Gromadzińsnka J, Wąsowicz W. (2014) Parabens. From environmental studies to human health. *Environment International.*

Bulzomi P, Bolli A, Galluzzo P, Acconcia F, Ascenzi P, Marino M. (2012) The naringenin-induced proapoptotic effect in breast cancer cell lines holds out against a high bisphenol a background. *International Union of Biochemistry and Molecular Biology Life.*

Byrne C, Divekar SD, Storchan GB, Parodi DA, Martin MB. (2013) Metals and breast cancer. *Journal of Mammary Gland Biology and Neoplasia.*

Chandran U, McCann SE, Zirpoli G, Gong Z, Lin Y, Hong CC, Ciupak G, Pawlish K, Ambrosone CB, Bandera EV. (2014) Intake of Energy-Dense Foods, Fast Foods, Sugary Drinks, and Breast Cancer Risk in African American and European American Women. *Nutrition and Cancer.*

Charles AK, Darbre PD. (2013) Combinations of parabens at concentrations measured in human breast tissue can increase proliferation of MCF-7 human breast cancer cells. *Journal of Applied Toxicology.*

Chen FP, Chien MH. (2014) Lower concentrations of phthalates induce proliferation in human breast cancer cells. *Climacteric.*

Chen M, Tao L, Collins EM, Austin C, Lu C. (2012) Simultaneous determination of multiple phthalate metabolites and bisphenol-A in human urine by liquid chromatography-tandem mass spectrometry. *Journal of Chromatography B Analytical Technologies in the Biomedical and Life Sciences.*

Crinnion WJ. (2010) Toxic effects of the easily avoidable phthalates and parabens. *Alternative Medicine Review.*

Dairkee SH, et al. (2008) Bisphenol A induces a profile of tumor aggressiveness in high-risk cells from breast cancer patients. *Cancer Research.*

Darbre PD. (2006) Metalloestrogens: an emerging class of inorganic xenoestrogens with potential to add to the estrogenic burden of the human breast. *Journal of Applied Toxicology.*

Darbre PD, Harvey PW. (2008) Paraben esters: review of recent studies of endocrine toxicity, absorption, esterase and human exposure, and discussion of potential human health risks. *Journal of Applied Toxicology.*

Darbre PD, Pugazhendhi D, Mannello F. (2011) Aluminum and human breast diseases. *Journal of Inorganic Biochemistry.*

Devi, G. (2014) BPA stimulates growth of an advanced subtype of human breast cancer cells called inflammatory breast cancer. *Endocrine Society.*

Egiebor E, Tulu A, Abou-Zeid N, Aighewi IT, Ishaque A. (2013) The kinetic signature of toxicity of four heavy metals and their mixtures on MCF7 breast cancer cell line. *International Journal of Environmental Research and Public Health.*

Fernandez SV, Huang Y, Snider KE, Zhou Y, Pogash TJ, Russo J. (2012) Expression and DNA methylation changes in human breast epithelial cells after bisphenol A exposure. *International Journal of Oncology.*

Frawley R, DeVito M, Walker NJ, Birnbaum L, White K Jr, Smith M, Maynor T, Recio L, Germolec D. (2014) Relative potency for altered humoral immunity induced by polybrominated and polychlorinated dioxins/furans in female B6C3F1/N mice. *Toxicological Sciences.*

Genuis SJ, Birkholz D, Curtis L, Sandau C. (2013) Paraben levels in an urban community of Western Canada. *ISRN Toxicology.*

Imran A, Engström A, Vahter M, Skerfving S, Lundh T, Lidfeldt J, Samsioe G, Halldin K, Åkesson A. (2014) Associations between cadmium exposure and circulating levels of sex hormones in postmenopausal women. *Environmental Research.*

Ishibe N, Hankinson SE, Colditz GA, Spiegelman D, Willett WC, Speizer FE, Kelsey KT, Hunter DJ. (1998) Cigarette smoking, cytochrome P450 1A1 polymorphisms, and breast cancer risk in the Nurses' Health Study. *Cancer Research.*

Khanna S, Dash PR, Darbre PD. (2014) Exposure to parabens at the concentration of maximal proliferative response increases migratory and invasive activity of human breast cancer cells in vitro. *Journal of Applied Toxicology.*

Kirchhof MG, de Gannes GC. (2013) The health controversies of parabens. *Skin Therapy Letter.*

Knower KC, To SQ, Leung YK, Ho SM, Clyne CD. (2014) Endocrine disruption of the epigenome: a breast cancer link. *Endocrine-Related Cancer.*

Konduracka E, Krzemieniecki K, Gajos G. (2014) Relationship between everyday use cosmetics and female breast cancer. *Polish Archives of Internal Medicine.*

Kotsopoulos J, et al. (2012) Plasma micronutrients, trace elements, and breast cancer in BRCA1 mutation carriers: an exploratory study. *Cancer Causes & Control.*

Kotsopoulos J, Sukiennicki G, Muszyńska M, Gackowski D, Kąklewski K, Durda K, Jaworska K, Huzarski T, Gronwald J, Byrski T, Ashuryk O, Dębniak T, Tołoczko-Grabarek A, Stawicka M, Godlewski D, Oliński R, Jakubowska A, Narod SA, Lubinski J. (2012) Plasma micronutrients, trace elements, and breast cancer in BRCA1 mutation carriers: an exploratory study. *Cancer Causes & Control.*

Lange C, Kuch B, Metzger JW. (2014) Estrogenic activity of constituents of underarm deodorants determined by E-Screen assay. *Chemosphere.*

López-Carrillo L, Hernández-Ramírez RU, Calafat AM, Torres-Sánchez L, Galván-Portillo M, Needham LL, Ruiz-Ramos R, Cebrián ME. (2010)

Exposure to phthalates and breast cancer risk in northern Mexico. *Environmental Health Perspectives.*

Mannello F, Ligi D, Canale M. (2013) Aluminum, carbonyls and cytokines in human nipple aspirate fluids: Possible relationship between inflammation, oxidative stress and breast cancer microenvironment. *Journal of Inorganic Biochemistry.*

Mervish N, McGovern KJ, Teitelbaum SL, Pinney SM, Windham GC, Biro FM, Kushi LH, Silva MJ, Ye X, Calafat AM, Wolff MS; BCERP. (2014) Dietary predictors of urinary environmental biomarkers in young girls, BCERP, 2004-7. *Environmental Research.*

Mohammadi M, Bakhtiari AR, Khodabandeh S. (2014) Concentration of cd, pb, hg, and se in different parts of human breast cancer tissues. *Journal of Toxicology.*

Nagata C, Nagao Y, Nakamura K, Wada K, Tamai Y, Tsuji M, Yamamoto S, Kashiki Y. (2013) Cadmium exposure and the risk of breast cancer in Japanese women. *Breast Cancer Research and Treatment.*

Nangia-Makker P, Raz T, Tait L, Shekhar MP, Li H, Balan V, Makker H, Fridman R, Maddipati K, Raz A. (2013) Ocimum gratissimum retards breast cancer growth and progression and is a natural inhibitor of matrix metalloproteases. *Cancer Biology & Therapy.*

Patterson AR, Mo X, Shapiro A, Wernke KE, Archer TK, Burd CJ. (2015) Sustained reprogramming of the estrogen response after chronic exposure to endocrine disruptors. *Molecular Endocrinology.*

Pazin M, Pereira LC, Dorta DJ. (2015) Toxicity of brominated flame retardants, BDE-47 and BDE-99 stems from impaired mitochondrial bioenergetics. *Toxicology Mechanisms and Methods.*

Pineau A, Fauconneau B, Sappino AP, Deloncle R, Guillard O. (2014) If exposure to aluminum in antiperspirants presents health risks, its content should be reduced. *Journal of Trace Elements in Medicine and Biology.*

Pluchino LA, Wang HCR. (2014) Chronic exposure to combined carcinogens enhances breast cell carcinogenesis with mesenchymal and stem-like cell properties. *PLoS One.*

Pupo M, Pisano A, Lappano R, Santolla MF, De Francesco EM, Abonante S, Rosano C, Maggiolini M. (2012) Bisphenol A Induces Gene Expression Changes and Proliferative Effects through GPER in

Breast Cancer Cells and Cancer-Associated Fibroblasts. *Environmental Health Perspectives.*

Romanowicz-Makowska H, Forma E, Bryś M, Krajewska WM, Smolarz B. (2011) Concentration of cadmium, nickel and aluminum in female breast cancer. *Polish Journal of Pathology.*

Saad H, Nasri I, Elwej A, Krayem N, Jarraya R, Kallel C, Zeghal N, Amara IB. (2014) A mineral and antioxidant-rich extract from the red marine Algae Alsidium corallinum exhibits cytoprotective effects against potassium bromate-induced erythrocyte oxidative damages in mice. *Biological Trace Element Research.*

Shenker NS, Polidoro S, van Veldhoven K, Sacerdote C, Ricceri F, Birrell MA, Belvisi MG, Brown R, Vineis P, Flanagan JM. (2013) Epigenome-wide association study in the European Prospective Investigation into Cancer and Nutrition (EPIC-Turin) identifies novel genetic loci associated with smoking. *Human Molecular Genetics.*

Singh S, Li SS. (2012) Epigenetic effects of environmental chemicals bisphenol a and phthalates. *International Journal of Molecular Sciences.*

Sundar S, Chakravarty J. (2010) Antimony Toxicity. *International Journal of Environmental Research and Public Health.*

Wittassek M, Koch HM, Angerer J, Brüning T. (2011) Assessing exposure to phthalates - the human biomonitoring approach. *Molecular Nutrition & Food Research.*

Wróbel AM, Gregoraszczuk EŁ. (2013) Effects of single and repeated in vitro exposure of three forms of parabens, methyl-, butyl- and propylparabens on the proliferation and estradiol secretion in MCF-7 and MCF-10A cells. *Pharmacological Reports.*

Wróbel AM, Gregoraszczuk EŁ. (2014) Differential effect of methyl-, butyl- and propylparaben and 17β-estradiol on selected cell cycle and apoptosis gene and protein expression in MCF-7 breast cancer cells and MCF-10A non-malignant cells. *Journal of Applied Toxicology.*

Wróbel AM, Gregoraszczuk EŁ. (2014) Actions of methyl-, propyl- and butylparaben on estrogen receptor-α and -β and the progesterone receptor in MCF-7 cancer cells and non-cancerous MCF-10A cells. *Toxicology Letters.*

Chapter Four: NUTRITION

Acharya A, Das I, Singh S, Saha T. (2010) Chemopreventive properties of indole-3-carbinol, diindolylmethane and other constituents of cardamom against carcinogenesis. *Recent Patents on Food, Nutrition and Agriculture.*

Adams LS, Kanaya N, Phung S, Liu Z, Chen S. (2011) Whole blueberry powder modulates the growth and metastasis of MDA-MB-231 triple negative breast tumors in nude mice. *Journal of Nutrition.*

Adams LS, Phung S, Yee N, Seeram NP, Li L, Chen S. (2010) Blueberry phytochemicals inhibit growth and metastatic potential of MDA-MB-231 breast cancer cells through modulation of the phosphatidylinositol 3-kinase pathway. *Cancer Research.*

Adebamowo CA, et al. (2005) Dietary flavonols and flavonol-rich foods intake and the risk of breast cancer. *International Journal of Cancer.*

Adhami VM, Khan N, Mukhtar H. (2009) Cancer chemoprevention by pomegranate: laboratory and clinical evidence. *Nutrition and Cancer.*

Adlercreutz H. (2010) Can rye intake decrease risk of human breast cancer? *Food & Nutrition Research.*

Aiyer HS, Warri AM, Woode DR, Hilakivi-Clarke L, Clarke R. (2012) Influence of berry polyphenols on receptor signaling and cell-death pathways: implications for breast cancer prevention. *Journal of Agricultural and Food Chemistry.*

Alfano CM, Imayama I, Neuhouser ML, Kiecolt-Glaser JK, Smith AW, Meeske K, McTiernan A, Bernstein L, Baumgartner KB, Ulrich CM, Ballard- Barbash R. (2012) Fatigue, inflammation, and ω-3 and ω-6 fatty acid intake among breast cancer survivors. *Journal of Clinical Oncology.*

Al-Ali KH, El-Beshbishy HA, El-Badry AA, Alkhalaf M. (2013) Cytotoxic activity of methanolic extract of Mentha longifolia and Ocimum basilicum against human breast cancer. *Pakistan Journal of Biological Sciences.*

Amrutha K, Nanjan P, Shaji SK, Sunilkumar D, Subhalakshmi K, Rajakrishna L, Banerji A. (2014) Discovery of lesser known flavones as inhibitors of NF-κB signaling in MDA-MB-231 breast cancer cells--A SAR study. *Bioorganic & Medicinal Chemistry Letters.*

Baharum Z, Akim AM, Taufiq-Yap YH, Hamid RA, Kasran R. (2014) In vitro antioxidant and antiproliferative activities of methanolic plant part extracts of Theobroma cacao. *Molecules.*

Bailly F, Toillon RA, Tomavo O, Jouy N, Hondermarck H, Cotelle P. (2013) Antiproliferative and apoptotic effects of the oxidative dimerization product of methyl caffeate on human breast cancer cells. *Bioorganic & Medicinal Chemistry Letters.*

Barrajón-Catalán E, Fernández-Arroyo S, Saura D, Guillén E, Fernández-Gutiérrez A, Segura-Carretero A, Micol V. (2010) Cistaceae aqueous extracts containing ellagitannins show antioxidant and antimicrobial capacity, and cytotoxic activity against human cancer cells. *Food and Chemical Toxicology.*

Bennett RN, Shiga TM, Hassimotto NM, Rosa EA, Lajolo FM, Cordenunsi BR. (2010) Phenolics and antioxidant properties of fruit pulp and cell wall fractions of postharvest banana (Musa acuminata Juss.) cultivars. *Journal of Agricultural and Food Chemistry.*

Berdowska I, Zieliński B, Fecka I, Kulbacka J, Saczko J, Gamian A. (2013) Cytotoxic impact of phenolics from Lamiaceae species on human breast cancer cells. *Food Chemistry.*

Berrino F, et al. (2006) Adjuvant diet to improve hormonal and metabolic factors affecting breast cancer prognosis. *Annals of the New York Academy of Sciences.*

Bhattacharya S, Ahir M, Patra P, Mukherjee S, Ghosh S, Mazumdar M, Chattopadhyay S, Das T, Chattopadhyay D, Adhikary A. (2015) PEGylated-thymoquinone-nanoparticle mediated retardation of breast cancer cell migration by deregulation of cytoskeletal actin polymerization through miR-34a. *Biomaterials.*

Bhui K, Tyagi S, Prakash B, Shukla Y. (2010) Pineapple bromelain induces autophagy, facilitating apoptotic response in mammary carcinoma cells. *BioFactors.*

Bhuvaneswari V, Nagini S. (2005) Lycopene: a review of its potential as an anticancer agent. *Current Medicinal Chemistry Anticancer Agents.*

Bougnoux, P. (2009) Improving outcome of chemotherapy of metastatic breast cancer by docosahexaenoic acid: a phase II trial. *British Journal of Cancer.*

Braicu C, Gherman CD, Irimie A, Berindan-Neagoe I. (2013) Epigallocatechin-3-Gallate (EGCG) inhibits cell proliferation and migratory behavior of triple negative breast cancer cells. *Journal of Nanoscience and Nanotechnology.*

Bulzomi P, Galluzzo P, Bolli A, Leone S, Acconcia F, Marino M. (2012) The pro-apoptotic effect of quercetin in cancer cell lines requires ERβ-dependent signals. *Journal of Cellular Physiology.*

Butalla AC, Crane TE, Patil B, Wertheim BC, Thompson P, Thomson CA. (2012) Effects of a carrot juice intervention on plasma carotenoids, oxidative stress, and inflammation in overweight breast cancer survivors. *Nutrition and Cancer.*

Caruso JA, Campana R, Wei C, Su CH, Hanks AM, Bornmann WG, Keyomarsi K. (2014) Indole-3-carbinol and its N-alkoxy derivatives preferentially target ERα-positive breast cancer cells. *Cell Cycle Research.*

Chandra-Kuntal K, Lee J, Singh SV. (2013) Critical role for reactive oxygen species in apoptosis induction and cell migration inhibition by diallyl trisulfide, a cancer chemopreventive component of garlic. *Breast Cancer Research and Treatment*

Chen Z, Zhang Y, et al. (2014) mTORC1/2 targeted by n-3 polyunsaturated fatty acids in the prevention of mammary tumorigenesis and tumor progression. *Oncogene.*

Chen HS, Bai MH, Zhang T, Li GD, Liu M. (2015) Ellagic acid induces cell cycle arrest and apoptosis through TGF-β/Smad3 signaling pathway in human breast cancer MCF-7 cells. *International Journal of Oncology.*

Collier RJ, et al. (2008) Effects of recombinant bovine somatotropin (rbST) and season on plasma and milk insulin-like growth factors I (IGF-I) and II (IGF-II) in lactating dairy cows. *Domestic Animal Endocrinology.*

Colomer R, Menéndez JA. (2006) Mediterranean diet, olive oil and cancer. *Clinical and Translational Oncology.*

Cordero-Herrera I, Martín MA, Goya L, Ramos S. (2015) Cocoa flavonoids protect hepatic cells function against high-glucose-induced oxidative stress: Relevance of MAPKs. *Molecular Nutrition & Food Research.*

Crew KD, et al. (2014) Effects of a green tea extract, Polyphenon E, on systemic biomarkers of growth factor signalling in women with hormone receptor-negative breast cancer. *Journal of Human Nutrition and Dietetics.*

Deandrea, S. (2008) Alcohol and breast cancer risk defined by estrogen and progesterone receptor status: a case–control study. *Cancer Epidemiology, Biomarkers & Prevention.*

Deguchi A. (2015) Curcumin targets in inflammation and cancer. *Endocrine, Metabolic & Immune Disorders Drug Targets.*

Dhandayuthapani S, Perez HD, Paroulek A, Chinnakkannu P, Kandalam U, Jaffe M, Rathinavelu A. (2012) Bromelain-induced apoptosis in GI-101A breast cancer cells. *Journal of Medicinal Food.*

Dinstel RR, Cascio J, Koukel S. (2013) The antioxidant level of Alaska's wild berries: high, higher and highest. *International Journal of Circumpolar Health.*

Do MT, Kim HG, Choi JH, Khanal T, Park BH, Tran TP, Jeong TC, Jeong HG. (2013) Antitumor efficacy of piperine in the treatment of human HER2-overexpressing breast cancer cells. *Food Chemistry.*

Donejko M, Niczyporuk M, Galicka E, Przylipiak A. (2013) Anticancer properties epigallocatechin-gallate contained in green tea. *Postępy Higieny i Medycyny Doświadczalnej.*

Dong Y, Cao A, Shi J, Yin P, Wang L, Ji G, Xie J, Wu D. (2014) Tangeretin, a citrus polymethoxyflavonoid, induces apoptosis of human gastric cancer AGS cells through extrinsic and intrinsic signaling pathways. *Oncology Reports.*

Drăgan, S. (2007) Role of multi-component functional foods in the complex treatment of patients with advanced breast cancer. *The Medical-Surgical Journal of the Society of Physicians and Naturalists Iasi, Romania.*

Duo J, Ying GG, Wang GW, Zhang L. (2012) Quercetin inhibits human breast cancer cell proliferation and induces apoptosis via Bcl-2 and Bax regulation. *Molecular Medicine Reports.*

Doucette CD, Hilchie AL, Liwski R, Hoskin DW. (2013) Piperine, a dietary phytochemical, inhibits angiogenesis. *The Journal of Nutritional Biochemistry.*

Einbond LS, Wu HA, Kashiwazaki R, He K, Roller M, Su T, Wang X, Goldsberry S. (2012) Carnosic acid inhibits the growth of ER-negative human breast cancer cells and synergizes with curcumin. *Fitoterapia.*

Eliassen AH, et al. (2012) Circulating carotenoids and risk of breast cancer: pooled analysis of eight prospective studies. *Journal of the National Cancer Institute.*

Ewaschuk JB, Newell M, Field CJ. (2012) Docosahexanoic Acid Improves Chemotherapy Efficacy by Inducing CD95 Translocation to Lipid Rafts in ER(-) Breast Cancer Cells. *Lipids.*

Farvid MS, Cho E, Chen WY, Eliassen AH, Willett WC. (2015) Adolescent meat intake and breast cancer risk. *International Journal of Cancer.*

Fowke JH. (2000) Brassica vegetable consumption shifts estrogen metabolism in healthy postmenopausal women. *Cancer Epidemiology, Biomarkers & Prevention.*

Fung TT, Chiuve SE, Willett WC, Hankinson SE, Hu FB, Holmes MD. (2013) Intake of specific fruits and vegetables in relation to risk of estrogen receptor-negative breast cancer among postmenopausal women. *Breast Cancer Research and Treatment.*

Galeone C. (2006) Onion and garlic use and human cancer. *American Journal of Clinical Nutrition.*

Gan FF, Ling H, Ang X, Reddy SA, Lee SS, Yang H, Tan SH, Hayes JD, Chui WK, Chew EH. (2013) A novel shogaol analog suppresses cancer cell invasion and inflammation, and displays cytoprotective effects through modulation of NF-κB and Nrf2-Keap1 signaling pathways. *Toxicology and Applied Pharmacology.*

Ganmaa, D. (2008) Coffee, tea, caffeine and risk of breast cancer: A 22-year follow-up. *International Journal of Cancer.*

García-Solís P, Yahia EM, Morales-Tlalpan V, Díaz-Muñoz M. (2009) Screening of antiproliferative effect of aqueous extracts of plant foods consumed in México on the breast cancer cell line MCF-7. *International Journal of Food Sciences and Nutrition.*

Gerhauser C. (2013) Epigenetic impact of dietary isothiocyanates in cancer chemoprevention. *Current Opinion in Clinical Nutrition and Metabolic Care.*

Gloria NF, Soares N, Brand C, Oliveira FL, Borojevic R, Teodoro AJ. (2014) Lycopene and beta-carotene induce cell-cycle arrest and apoptosis in human breast cancer cell lines. *Anticancer Research.*

González-Vallinas M, Molina S, Vicente G, Sánchez-Martínez R, Vargas T, García-Risco MR, Fornari T, Reglero G, Ramírez de Molina A. (2014) Modulation of estrogen and epidermal growth factor receptors by rosemary extract in breast cancer cells. *Electrophoresis.*

Grant WB. (2008) An ecological study of cancer mortality rates including indices for dietary iron and zinc. *Anticancer Research.*

Gu JW, Makey KL, Tucker KB, Chinchar E, Mao X, Pei I, Thomas EY, Miele L. (2013) EGCG, a major green tea catechin suppresses breast tumor angiogenesis and growth via inhibiting the activation of HIF-1α and NFκB, and VEGF expression. *Vascular Cell.*

Gunter MJ, et al. (2009) Insulin, insulin-like growth factor-I, and risk of breast cancer in postmenopausal women. *Journal of the National Cancer Institute.*

Hardman WE. (2014) Walnuts have potential for cancer prevention and treatment in mice. *Journal of Nutrition.*

Hattori M, Kawakami K, Akimoto M, Takenaga K, Suzumiya J, Honma Y. (2013) Antitumor effect of Japanese apricot extract (MK615) on human cancer cells in vitro and in vivo through a reactive oxygen species-dependent mechanism. *Tumori.*

He X, Wang Y, Hu H, Zhang Z. (2012) In vitro and in vivo antimammary tumor activities and mechanisms of the apple total triterpenoids. *Journal of Agricultural and Food Chemistry.*

Hou DX. (2003) Potential mechanisms of cancer chemoprevention by anthocyanins. *Current Molecular Medicine.*

Huang C, Lee SY, Lin CL, Tu TH, Chen LH, Chen YJ, Huang HC. (2013) Co-treatment with quercetin and 1,2,3,4,6-penta-O-galloyl-β-D-glucose causes cell cycle arrest and apoptosis in human breast cancer MDA-MB-231 and AU565 cells. *Journal of Agricultural and Food Chemistry.*

Huang WY, Cai YZ, Zhang Y (2010) Natural phenolic compounds from medicinal herbs and dietary plants: potential use for cancer prevention. *Nutrition and Cancer.*

Hudson EA, et al. (2000) Characterization of potentially chemopreventive phenols in extracts of brown rice that inhibit the growth of human breast and colon cancer cells. *Cancer Epidemiology, Biomarkers & Prevention.*

Jabri Karoui I, Marzouk B. (2013) Characterization of bioactive compounds in Tunisian bitter orange (Citrus aurantium L.) peel and juice and determination of their antioxidant activities. *BioMed Research International.*

Jafarian-Dehkordi A, Zolfaghari B, Mirdamadi M. (2013) The effects of chloroform, ethyl acetate and methanolic extracts of Brassica rapa L. on cell-mediated immune response in mice. *Research in Pharmaceutical Sciences.*

Johnson JJ. (2011) Carnosol: a promising anticancer and anti-inflammatory agent. *Cancer Letters.*

Jordan I, Hebestreit A, Swai B, Krawinkel MB. (2013) Dietary patterns and breast cancer risk among women in northern Tanzania: a case-control study. *European Journal of Nutrition.*

Kanazawa K, Sakakibara H. (2000) High content of dopamine, a strong antioxidant, in Cavendish banana. *Journal of Agricultural and Food Chemistry.*

Kim ND. (2002) Chemopreventive and adjuvant therapeutic potential of pomegranate (Punica granatum) for human breast cancer. *Breast Cancer Research and Treatment.*

Kim, YI. (2006) Does a high folate intake increase the risk of breast cancer? *Nutrition Reviews.*

Krone CA, Ely JT. (2005) Controlling hyperglycemia as an adjunct to cancer therapy. *Integrative Cancer Therapies.*

Lan T, Wang L, Xu Q, Liu W, Jin H, Mao W, Wang X, Wang X. (2013) Growth inhibitory effect of Cucurbitacin E on breast cancer cells. *International Journal of Clinical and Experimental Pathology.*

Larsson SC, Bergkvist L, Wolk A. (2010) Dietary carotenoids and risk of hormone receptor-defined breast cancer in a prospective cohort of Swedish women. *European Journal of Cancer.*

Lea MA. (2015) Flavonol Regulation in Tumor Cells. *Journal of Cellular Biochemistry.*

Lee SA, et al. (2008) Cruciferous vegetables, the GSTP1 Ile105Val genetic polymorphism, and breast cancer risk. *American Journal of Clinical Nutrition.*

Lee CJ, et al. (2010) Hesperidin suppressed proliferations of both human breast cancer and androgen-dependent prostate cancer cells. *Phytotherapy Research.*

Lew JQ. (2009) Alcohol and risk of breast cancer by histologic type and hormone receptor status in postmenopausal women: the NIH-AARP Diet and Health Study. *American Journal of Epidemiology.*

Li H, Yang B, Huang J, Xiang T, Yin X, Wan J, Luo F, Zhang L, Li H, Ren G. (2013) Naringin inhibits growth potential of human triple-negative breast cancer cells by targeting β-catenin signaling pathway. *Toxicology Letters.*

Licznerska BE, Szaefer H, Murias M, Bartoszek A, Baer-Dubowska W. (2013) Modulation of CYP19 expression by cabbage juices and their active components: indole-3-carbinol and 3,3'-diindolylmethene in human breast epithelial cell lines. *European Journal of Nutrition.*

Lirdprapamongkol K, Sakurai H, Kawasaki N, Choo MK, Saitoh Y, Aozuka Y, Singhirunnusorn P, Ruchirawat S, Svasti J, Saiki I. (2005) Vanillin suppresses in vitro invasion and in vivo metastasis of mouse breast cancer cells. *European Journal of Pharmaceutical Sciences.*

Liu J, Ma DW. (2014) The role of n-3 polyunsaturated fatty acids in the prevention and treatment of breast cancer. *Nutrients.*

López-Carillo L, Hernández-Ramirez RU, Calafat AM, Torres-Sánchez L, Galván-Portillo M, Needham LL, Ruiz-Ramos R, Cebriáan ME. (2010) Exposure to phthalates and breast cancer risk in northern Mexico. *Environmental Health Perspectives.*

Luo J, Gao YT, Chow WH, Shu XO, Li H, Yang G, Cai Q, Li G, Rothman N, Cai H, Shrubsole MJ, Franke AA, Zheng W, Dai Q. (2012) Urinary polyphenols, glutathione S-transferases copy number variation, and breast cancer risk: results from the Shanghai women's health study. *Molecular Carcinogenesis.*

Maeda N. (2007) Inhibitory effect on replicative DNA polymerases, human cancer cell proliferation, and in vivo anti-tumor activity by glycolipids from spinach. *Current Medicinal Chemistry.*

Majdalawieh AF, Carr RI. (2010). In Vitro Investigation of the Potential Immunomodulatory and Anticancer Activities of Black Pepper (Piper nigrum) and Cardamom (Elettaria cardamomum). *Journal of Medicinal Food.*

Mak KK, Wu AT, Lee WH, Chang TC, Chiou JF, Wang LS, Wu CH, Huang CY, Shieh YS, Chao TY, Ho CT, Yen GC, Yeh CT. (2013) Pterostilbene, a bioactive component of blueberries, suppresses the generation of breast cancer stem cells within tumor microenvironment and metastasis via modulating NF-κB/microRNA 448 circuit. *Molecular Nutrition & Food Research.*

Maroof H, Hassan ZM, Mobarez AM, Mohamadabadi MA. (2012) Lactobacillus acidophilus could modulate the immune response against breast cancer in murine model. *Journal of Clinical Immunology.*

Marques M, Laflamme L, Benassou I, Cissokho C, Guillemette B, Gaudreau L. (2014) Low levels of 3,3'-diindolylmethane activate estrogen receptor α and induce proliferation of breast cancer cells in the absence of estradiol. *BioMed Central Cancer.*

Martin KR, Wooden A. (2012) Tart Cherry Juice Induces Differential Dose-Dependent Effects on Apoptosis, But Not Cellular Proliferation, in MCF-7 Human Breast Cancer Cells. *Journal of Medicinal Food.*

Mason JK, Thompson LU. (2014) Flaxseed and its lignan and oil components: can they play a role in reducing the risk of and improving the treatment of breast cancer? *Applied Physiology, Nutrition, and Metabolism.*

Matkowski A, Kuś P, Góralska E, Woźniak D. (2013) Mangiferin - a bioactive xanthonoid, not only from mango and not just antioxidant. *Mini-Reviews in Medicinal Chemistry.*

Mignone LI, et al. (2009) Dietary carotenoids and the risk of invasive breast cancer. *International Journal of Cancer.*

Miller JA, Lang JE, Ley M, Nagle R, Hsu CH, Thompson PA, Cordova C, Waer A, Chow HH. (2013) Human breast tissue disposition and bioactivity of limonene in women with early-stage breast cancer. *Cancer Prevention Research (Philadelphia).*

Milner JA. (2006) Preclinical Perspectives on Garlic and Cancer. *Journal of Nutrition.*

Modem S, Dicarlo SE, Reddy TR. (2012) Fresh Garlic Extract Induces Growth Arrest and Morphological Differentiation of MCF7 Breast Cancer Cells. *Genes & Cancer.*

Munagala R, Aqil F, Vadhanam MV, Gupta RC. (2013) MicroRNA 'signature' during estrogen-mediated mammary carcinogenesis and its reversal by ellagic acid intervention. *Cancer Letters.*

Nangia-Makker P, Raz T, Tait L, Shekhar MP, Li H, Balan V, Makker H, Fridman R, Maddipati K, Raz A. (2013) Ocimum gratissimum retards breast cancer growth and progression and is a natural inhibitor of matrix metalloproteases. *Cancer Biology & Therapy.*

Ngo SN, Williams DB, Head RJ. (2011) Rosemary and cancer prevention: preclinical perspectives. *Critical Reviews in Food Science and Nutrition.*

Nicastro HL, Firestone GL, Bjeldanes LF. (2013) 3,3'-diindolylmethane rapidly and selectively inhibits hepatocyte growth factor/c-Met signaling in breast cancer cells. *Journal of Nutritional Biochemistry.*

Onodera Y, Nam JM, Bissell MJ. (2014) Increased sugar uptake promotes oncogenesis via EPAC/RAP1 and O-GlcNAc pathways. *American Society for Clinical Investigation - Journal of Clinical Investigation.*

Okic-Djordjevic I, Trivanovic D, Krstic J, Jaukovic A, Mojsilovic S, Santibanez JF, Terzic M, Vesovic D, Bugarski D. (2013) GE132+Natural: Novel promising dietetic supplement with antiproliferative influence on prostate, colon, and breast cancer cells. *The Journal of Balkan Union of Oncology.*

Oleaga C, García M, Solé A, Ciudad CJ, Izquierdo-Pulido M, Noé V. (2012) CYP1A1 is overexpressed upon incubation of breast cancer cells with a polyphenolic cocoa extract. *European Journal of Nutrition.*

Olsson ME, et al. (2004). Inhibition of cancer cell proliferation in vitro by fruit and berry extracts and correlations with antioxidant levels. *Journal of Agricultural and Food Chemistry.*

Pandurangan AK, Saadatdoust Z, Mohd Esa N, Hamzah H, Ismail A. (2015) Dietary cocoa protects against colitis-associated cancer by activating the Nrf2/Keap1 pathway. *Biofactors.*

Park JH, Lee MK, Yoon J. (2015) Gamma-linolenic acid inhibits hepatic PAI-1 expression by inhibiting p38 MAPK-dependent activator protein and mitochondria-mediated apoptosis pathway. *Apoptosis.*

Pouchieu C, Galan P, Ducros V, Latino-Martel P, Hercberg S, Touvier M. (2014) Plasma carotenoids and retinol and overall and breast cancer risk: a nested case-control study. *Nutrition and Cancer.*

Radwan AA, Alanazi FK, Al-Dhfyan A. (2013) Synthesis, and docking studies of some fused-quinazolines and quinazolines carrying biological active isatin moiety as cell-cycle inhibitors of breast cancer cell lines. *Drug Research.*

Ramljak D, Romanczyk LJ, Metheny-Barlow LJ, Thompson N, Knezevic V, Galperin M, Ramesh A, Dickson RB. (2005) Pentameric procyanidin from Theobroma cacao selectively inhibits growth of human breast cancer cells. *Molecular Cancer Therapeutics.*

Ravoori S, Vadhanam MV, Aqil F, Gupta RC. (2012) Inhibition of estrogen-mediated mammary tumorigenesis by blueberry and black raspberry. *Journal of Agricultural and Food Chemistry.*

Reagan-Shaw S, Eggert D, Mukhtar H, Ahmad N. (2010) Antiproliferative effects of apple peel extract against cancer cells. *Nutrition and Cancer.*

Ribaya-Mercado JD, et al. (2004) Lutein and zeaxanthin and their potential roles in disease prevention. *Journal of American College of Nutrition.*

Ricceri F et al. (2015) Risk of second primary malignancies in women with breast cancer: Results from the European Prospective Investigation into Cancer and Nutrition (EPIC). *International Journal of Cancer.*

Rocha A, Wang L, Penichet M, Martins-Green M. (2012) Pomegranate juice and specific components inhibit cell and molecular processes critical for metastasis of breast cancer. *Breast Cancer Research and Treatment.*

Rock CL, et al. (2005). Plasma carotenoids and recurrence-free survival in women with a history of breast cancer. *Journal of Clinical Oncology.*

Rodríguez-Cruz, M. (2005) Molecular mechanisms of action and health benefits of polyunsaturated fatty acids. *Journal of Clinical Investigations.*

Sae-Teaw M, Johns J, Johns NP, Subongkot S. (2013) Serum melatonin levels and antioxidant capacities after consumption of pineapple, orange, or banana by healthy male volunteers. *Journal of Pineal Research.*

Sangai NP, Verma RJ, Trivedi MH. (2014) Testing the efficacy of quercetin in mitigating bisphenol A toxicity in liver and kidney of mice. *Toxicology and Industrial Health.*

Santana-Rios G. (2001) Potent antimutagenic activity of white tea in comparison with green tea in the Salmonella assay. *Mutation Research.*

Seeram NP. (2006) Blackberry, black raspberry, blueberry, cranberry, red raspberry, and strawberry extracts inhibit growth and stimulate apoptosis of human cancer cells in vitro. *Journal of Agricultural and Food Chemistry.*

Shi ZY, Li YQ, Kang YH, Hu GQ, Huang-fu CS, Deng JB, Liu B. (2012) Piperonal ciprofloxacin hydrazone induces growth arrest and apoptosis of human hepatocarcinoma SMMC-7721 cells. *Journal of the Chinese Pharmacological Society.*

Shike M, et al. (2014) The Effects of Soy Supplementation on Gene Expression in Breast Cancer: A Randomized Placebo-Controlled Study. *Journal of the National Cancer Institute.*

Sieri S, et al. (2008) Dietary fat and breast cancer risk in the European Prospective Investigation into Cancer and Nutrition. *American Journal of Clinical Nutrition.*

Slavin J. (2013) Fiber and prebiotics: mechanisms and health benefits. *Nutrients.*

Somasagara RR, Hegde M, Chiruvella KK, Musini A, Choudhary B, Raghavan SC. (2012) Extracts of strawberry fruits induce intrinsic pathway of apoptosis in breast cancer cells and inhibits tumor progression in mice. *PLoS One.*

Song NR, Chung MY, Kang NJ, Seo SG, Jang TS, Lee HJ, Lee KW. (2014) Quercetin suppresses invasion and migration of H-Ras-transformed MCF10A human epithelial cells by inhibiting phosphatidylinositol 3-kinase. *Food Chemistry.*

Suez J, et al. (2014) Artificial sweeteners induce glucose intolerance by altering the gut microbiota. *Nature.*

Sun T, Chen QY, Wu LJ, Yao XM, Sun XJ. (2012) Antitumor and antimetastatic activities of grape skin polyphenols in a murine model of breast cancer. *Food and Chemical Toxicology.*

Suzuki R, et al. (2008) Dietary lignans and postmenopausal breast cancer risk by estrogen receptor status: a prospective cohort study of Swedish women. *British Journal of Cancer.*

Szaefer H, Licznerska B, Krajka-Kuźniak V, Bartoszek A, Baer-Dubowska W. (2012) Modulation of CYP1A1, CYP1A2 and CYP1B1 expression by cabbage juices and indoles in human breast cell lines. *Nutrition and Cancer.*

Takeda S, Okajima S, Miyoshi H, Yoshida K, Okamoto Y, Okada T, Amamoto T, Watanabe K, Omiecinski CJ, Aramaki H. (2012) Cannabidiolic acid, a major cannabinoid in fiber-type cannabis, is an inhibitor of MDA-MB-231 breast cancer cell migration. *Toxicology Letters.*

Tamimi RM, et al. (2009) Circulating carotenoids, mammographic density, and subsequent risk of breast cancer. *Cancer Research.*

Tanaka T, Tanaka T, Tanaka M, Kuno T. (2012) Cancer chemoprevention by citrus pulp and juices containing high amounts of β-cryptoxanthin and hesperidin. *Journal of Biomedicine and Biotechnology.*

Tang EL, Rajarajeswaran J, Fung SY, Kanthimathi MS. (2013) Antioxidant activity of Coriandrum sativum and protection against DNA damage and cancer cell migration. *BMC Complementary and Alternative Medicine.*

Tarko T, Duda-Chodak A, Zajac N. (2013) Digestion and absorption of phenolic compounds assessed by in vitro simulation methods. *Roczniki Państwowego Zakładu Higieny.*

Taylor EF, et al. (2007) Meat consumption and risk of breast cancer in the UK Women's Cohort Study. *British Journal of Cancer.*

Taylor VH, et al. (2009) Is red meat intake a risk factor for breast cancer among premenopausal women? *Breast Cancer Research and Treatment.*

Thomson CA, et al. (2007) Plasma and dietary carotenoids are associated with reduced oxidative stress in women previously treated for breast cancer. *Cancer Epidemiology, Biomarkers & Prevention.*

Thompson LU, et al. (2005) Dietary flaxseed alters tumor biological markers in postmenopausal breast cancer. *Clinical Cancer Research.*

Tin AS, Park AH, Sundar SN, Firestone GL. (2014) Essential role of the cancer stem/progenitor cell marker nucleostemin for indole-3-carbinol anti-proliferative responsiveness in human breast cancer cells. *BioMed Central Biology.*

Trejo-Solís C, Pedraza-Chaverrí J, Torres-Ramos M, Jiménez-Farfán D, Cruz Salgado A, Serrano-García N, Osorio-Rico L, Sotelo J. (2013) Multiple molecular and cellular mechanisms of action of lycopene in cancer inhibition. *Evidence-Based Complementary and Alternative Medicine.*

Tyagi T, Treas JN, Mahalingaiah PK, Singh KP. (2015) Potentiation of growth inhibition and epigenetic modulation by combination of green tea polyphenol and 5-aza-2'-deoxycytidine in human breast cancer cells. *Breast Cancer Research and Treatment.*

Velentzis LS, et al. (2009) Lignans and breast cancer risk in pre- and post-menopausal women: meta-analyses of observational studies. *British Journal of Cancer.*

Vicennati V, Garelli S, Rinaldi E, Rosetti S, Zavatta G, Pagotto U, Pasquali R. (2015) Obesity-related proliferative diseases: the interaction between adipose tissue and estrogens in post-menopausal women. *Hormone Molecular Biology and Clinical Investigation Journal.*

Vidhya N, Devaraj SN. (2011) Induction of apoptosis by eugenol in human breast cancer cells. *Indian Journal of Experimental Biology.*

Virk-Baker MK, Barnes S, Krontiras H, Nagy TR. (2014) S-(-)equol producing status not associated with breast cancer risk among low isoflavone-consuming US postmenopausal women undergoing a physician-recommended breast biopsy. *Nutrition Research.*

Viry E, Anwar A, Kirsch G, Jacob C, Diederich M, Bagrel D. (2011) Antiproliferative effect of natural tetrasulfides in human breast cancer cells is mediated through the inhibition of the cell division cycle 25 phosphatases. *International Journal of Oncology.*

Vizzotto M, Porter W, Byrne D, Cisneros-Zevallos L. (2014) Polyphenols of selected peach and plum genotypes reduce cell viability and inhibit proliferation of breast cancer cells while not affecting normal cells. *Food Chemistry.*

Xia Y, et al. (2007) The potentiation of curcumin on insulin-like growth factor-1 action in MCF-7 human breast carcinoma cells. *Life Sciences.*

Xue M, Wang Q, Zhao J, Dong L, Ge Y, Hou L, Liu Y, Zheng Z. (2014) Docosahexaenoic acid inhibited the Wnt/β-catenin pathway and suppressed breast cancer cells in vitro and in vivo. *Journal of Nutritional Biochemistry.*

Yamazaki S, Miyoshi N, Kawabata K, Yasuda M, Shimoi K. (2014) Quercetin-3-O-glucuronide inhibits noradrenaline-promoted invasion of MDA-MB-231 human breast cancer cells by blocking β_2-adrenergic signaling. *Archives of Biochemistry and Biophysiology.*

Yang D, et al. (2013) Dietary Intake of Folate, B-Vitamins and Methionine and Breast Cancer Risk among Hispanic and Non-Hispanic White Women. *PLoS One.*

Yesil-Celiktas O, Sevimli C, Bedir E, Vardar-Sukan F. (2010) Inhibitory effects of rosemary extracts, carnosic acid and rosmarinic acid on the growth of various human cancer cell lines. *Plant Foods and Human Nutrition.*

Yiannakopoulou EC. (2014) Effect of green tea catechins on breast carcinogenesis: a systematic review of in-vitro and in-vivo experimental studies. *European Journal of Cancer Prevention.*

Yiannakopoulou EC. (2014) Green Tea Catechins: Proposed Mechanisms of Action in Breast Cancer Focusing on the Interplay Between Survival and Apoptosis. *Anticancer Agents in Medicinal Chemistry.*

Yu MH. (2007) Induction of apoptosis by immature fruits of Prunus salicina Lindl. cv. Soldam in MDA-MB-231 human breast cancer cells. *International Journal of Food Sciences and Nutrition.*

Zheng JS, Hu XJ, Zhao YM, Yang J, Li D. (2013) Intake of fish and marine n-3 polyunsaturated fatty acids and risk of breast cancer: meta-analysis of data from 21 independent prospective cohort studies. *British Medical Journal.*

Zheng W, Lee SA. (2009) Well-done meat intake, heterocyclic amine exposure, and cancer risk. *Nutrition and Cancer.*

Chapter Five: MICROBIAL HEALTH

Alcock J, Maley CC, Aktipis CA. (2014) Is eating behavior manipulated by the gastrointestinal microbiota? Evolutionary pressures and potential mechanisms. *Bioessays.*

Aragón F, Carino S, Perdigón G, de Moreno de LeBlanc A. (2014) The administration of milk fermented by the probiotic Lactobacillus casei CRL 431 exerts an immunomodulatory effect against a breast tumor in a mouse model. *Immunobiology.*

Aragón F, Perdigón G, de Moreno de LeBlanc A. (2014) Modification in the diet can induce beneficial effects against breast cancer. *World Journal of Clinical Oncology.*

Kaetzel CS. (2014) Cooperativity among secretory IgA, the polymeric immunoglobulin receptor, and the gut microbiota promotes host-microbial mutualism. *Immunology Letters.*

Kaga C, Takagi A, Kano M, Kado S, Kato I, Sakai M, Miyazaki K, Nanno M, Ishikawa F, Ohashi Y, Toi M. (2013) Lactobacillus casei Shirota enhances the preventive efficacy of soymilk in chemically induced breast cancer. *Cancer Science.*

Kassayová M, Bobrov N, Strojný L, Kisková T, Mikeš J, Demečková V, Orendáš P, Bojková B, Péč M, Kubatka P, Bomba A. (2014) Preventive effects of probiotic bacteria Lactobacillus plantarum and dietary fiber in chemically-induced mammary carcinogenesis. *Anticancer Research.*

Lakritz JR, Poutahidis T, Levkovich T, Varian BJ, Ibrahim YM, Chatzigiagkos A, Mirabal S, Alm EJ, Erdman SE. (2014) Beneficial bacteria stimulate host immune cells to counteract dietary and genetic predisposition to mammary cancer in mice. *International Journal of Cancer.*

Maroof H, Hassan ZM, Mobarez AM, Mohamadabadi MA. (2012) Lactobacillus acidophilus could modulate the immune response against breast cancer in murine model. *Journal of Clinical Immunology.*

Nackerdien ZE. (2008) Perspectives on microbes as oncogenic infectious agents and implications for breast cancer. *Medical Hypotheses.*

Shapira I, Sultan K, Lee A, Taioli E. (2013) Evolving Concepts: How Diet and the Intestinal Microbiome Act as Modulators of Breast Malignancy. *ISRN Oncology.*

Urbaniak C, Cummins J, Brackstone M, Macklaim JM, Gloor GB, Baban CK, Scott L, O'Hanlon DM, Burton JP, Francis KP, Tangney M, Reid G. (2014) Bacterial microbiota of human breast tissue. *Applied and Environmental Microbiology.*

Wink M, Ashour ML, El-Readi MZ. (2012) Secondary Metabolites from Plants Inhibiting ABC Transporters and Reversing Resistance of Cancer Cells and Microbes to Cytotoxic and Antimicrobial Agents. *Frontiers in Microbiology.*

Xuan C, Shamonki JM, Chung A, Dinome ML, Chung M, Sieling PA, Lee DJ. (2014) Microbial dysbiosis is associated with human breast cancer. *PLoS One.*

Chapter Six: SUPPLEMENTS

Bolhassani A. (2015) Cancer chemoprevention by natural carotenoids as an efficient strategy. *Anticancer Agents in Medicinal Chemistry.*

Cann SA, van Netten JP, van Netten C. (2000) Hypothesis: iodine, selenium and the development of breast cancer. *Cancer Causes & Control.*

Castillo-L C, Tur JA, Uauy R. (2012) Folate and breast cancer risk: a systematic review. *Revista médica de Chile.*

Cooney RV, Dai Q, Gao YT, Chow WH, Franke AA, Shu XO, Li H, Ji B, Cai Q, Chai W, Zheng W. (2011) Low plasma coenzyme Q(10) levels and breast cancer risk in Chinese women. *Cancer Epidemiology, Biomarkers & Prevention.*

Chu XT, Dela Cruz J, Hwang SG, Hong H. (2014) Tumorigenic Effects of Endocrine-Disrupting Chemicals are Alleviated by Licorice (Glycyrrhiza glabra) Root Extract through Suppression of AhR Expression in Mammalian Cells. *Asian Pacific Journal of Cancer Prevention.*

de Campos-Ferraz PL, Andrade I, das Neves W, Hangai I, Alves CR, Lancha Jr AH. (2014) An overview of amines as nutritional supplements to counteract cancer cachexia. *Journal of Cachexia, Sarcopenia and Muscle.*

Duo J, Ying GG, Wang GW, Zhang L. (2012) Quercetin inhibits human breast cancer cell proliferation and induces apoptosis via Bcl-2 and Bax regulation. *Molecular Medicine Report.*

Gombart AF, Luong QT, Koeffler HP. (2006) Vitamin D compounds: activity against microbes and cancer. *Anticancer Research.*

Grant SG, et al. (2009) Melatonin and breast cancer: cellular mechanisms, clinical studies and future perspectives. *Expert Reviews in Molecular Medicine.*

Greenlee H, Shaw J, Lau YK, Naini A, Maurer M. (2012) Lack of effect of coenzyme q10 on Doxorubicin cytotoxicity in breast cancer cell cultures. *Integrative Cancer Therapy.*

Haim A, Zubidat AE. (2015) Artificial light at night: melatonin as a mediator between the environment and epigenome. *Philosophical Transactions of the Royal Society of London B Biological Sciences.*

Hilakivi-Clarke L. (2004). Nutritional modulation of the cell cycle and breast cancer. *Endocrine-Related Cancer.*

Jung B, Ahmad N. (2006) Melatonin in cancer management: progress and promise. *Cancer Research.*

Kidd P. (1996) A New Approach to Metastatic Cancer Prevention: Modified Citrus Pectin (MCP), A Unique pectin that Blocks Cell Surface Lectins. *Alternative Medicine Review.*

Kim Y. (2006) Does a high folate intake increase the risk of breast cancer? *Nutrition Reviews.*

Kondegowda NG, Meaney MP, Baker C, Ju YH. (2011) Effects of non-digestible carbohydrates on the growth of estrogen-dependent human breast cancer (MCF-7) tumors implanted in ovariectomized athymic mice. *Nutrition and Cancer.*

Lance J, McCabe S, Clancy RL, Pierce J. (2012) Coenzyme Q10--a therapeutic agent. *Medical-Surgical Nursing.*

Li M, Chen P, Li J, Chu R, Xie D, Wang H. (2014) Review: the impacts of circulating 25-hydroxyvitamin d levels on cancer patient outcomes: a systematic review and meta-analysis. *Journal of Clinical Endocrinology and Metabolism.*

Lockwood K, Moesgaard S, Hanioka T, Folkers K. (1994) Apparent partial remission of breast cancer in 'high risk' patients supplemented with nutritional antioxidants, essential fatty acids and coenzyme Q10. *Molecular Aspects of Medicine.*

Martínez-Campa CM, Alonso-González C, Mediavilla MD, Cos S, González A, Sanchez-Barcelo EJ. (2008) Melatonin down-regulates hTERT expression induced by either natural estrogens (17beta-estradiol) or metalloestrogens (cadmium) in MCF-7 human breast cancer cells. *Cancer Letters.*

Nangia-Makker P, Hogan V, Honjo Y, Baccarini S, Tait L, Bresalier R, Raz A. (2002) Inhibition of human cancer cell growth and metastasis in nude mice by oral intake of modified citrus pectin. *Journal of the National Cancer Institute.*

Obaidi J, Musallam E, Al-Ghzawi HM, Azzeghaiby SN, Alzoghaibi IN. (2014) Vitamin D and its relationship with breast cancer: an evidence based practice paper. *Global Journal of Health Sciences.*

Patrick L. (2008) Iodine: deficiency and therapeutic considerations. *Alternative Medicine Review.*

Premkumar VG, et al. (2007) Serum cytokine levels of interleukin-1β,-6, -8, tumour necrosis factor-α and vascular endothelial growth factor in breast cancer patients treated with tamoxifen and supplemented with co-enzyme Q(10), riboflavin and niacin. *Basic Clinical Pharmacology & Toxicology.*

Reid ME. (2008) The nutritional prevention of cancer: 400 mcg per day selenium treatment. *Nutrition and Cancer.*

Schrauzer GN. (2009) Selenium and selenium-antagonistic elements in nutritional cancer prevention. *Critical Review in Biotechnology.*

Xiao X, Shi D, Liu L, Wang J, Xie X, Kang T, Deng W. (2011) Quercetin suppresses cyclooxygenase-2 expression and angiogenesis through inactivation of P300 signaling. *PLoS One.*

Xiaorui L, et al. (2012) Carotenoids Play a Positive Role in the Degradation of Heteroclyles by Sphingobium yanoikuyae. *PLoS One.*

Yuvaraj S. (2008) Augmented antioxidant status in Tamoxifen treated postmenopausal women with breast cancer on co-administration with

Coenzyme Q10, Niacin and Riboflavin. *Cancer Chemotherapy and Pharmacology.*

Chapter Seven: SELF–CARE

Blask DE, Dauchy RT, Dauchy EM, Mao L, Hill SM, Greene MW, Belancio VP, Sauer LA, Davidson L. (2014) Light exposure at night disrupts host/ cancer circadian regulatory dynamics: impact on the Warburg effect, lipid signaling and tumor growth prevention. *PLoS One.*

Dauchy RT, Xiang S, Mao L, Brimer S, Wren MA, Yuan L, Anbalagan M, Hauch A, Frasch T, Rowan BG, Blask DE, Hill SM. (2014) Circadian and melatonin disruption by exposure to light at night drives intrinsic resistance to tamoxifen therapy in breast cancer. *Cancer Research.*

Dobos G, Overhamm T, Büssing A, Ostermann T, Langhorst J, Kümmel S, Paul A, Cramer H. (2015) Integrating mindfulness in supportive cancer care: a cohort study on a mindfulness-based day care clinic for cancer survivors. *Supportive Care in Cancer.*

Ghose A, Kundu R, Toumeh A, Hornbeck C, Mohamed I. (2015) A Review of Obesity, Insulin Resistance, and the Role of Exercise in Breast Cancer Patients. *Nutrition and Cancer.*

Leung N, Furniss D, Giele H. (2015) Modern surgical management of breast cancer therapy related upper limb and breast lymphoedema. *Maturitas.*

Malina C. Frigo S, Mathelin C. (2013) Sleep and breast cancer: Is there a link? *Gynecology, Obstetrics and Fertility.*

Rabstein S, et al. (2014) Polymorphisms in circadian genes, night work and breast cancer: results from the GENICA study. *Chronobiology International Journal.*

Stevens RG, Zhu Y. (2015) Electric light, particularly at night, disrupts human circadian rhythmicity: is that a problem? *Philosophical Transactions of the Royal Society of London Series B Biological Sciences.*

Swisher AK, Abraham J, Bonner D, Gilleland D, Hobbs G, Kurian S, Yanosik MA, Vona-Davis L. (2015) Exercise and dietary advice intervention for survivors of triple-negative breast cancer: effects on body fat, physical function, quality of life, and adipokine profile. *Supportive Care in Cancer.*

GLOSSARIES

Anyone dealing with cancer can quickly become medically literate, as it is necessary to understand the terms used by doctors and medical researchers. To fully understand the research that supports the current functional medicine recommendations for breast cancer patients, we need to also understand terms used to describe metabolism, nutrition, toxins, genetics, and statistics. No one can be expected to be fluent in all of the areas of science that are interwoven throughout this book. Therefore, this section provides two extensive glossaries that define the terms that may be unfamiliar. Using the proper terminology is often the clearest way to explain a scientific concept.

The first glossary covers medical and technical terminology. The second covers nutrients and nutrition terminology.

Glossary of Medical and Technical Terms

Adipose—medical term for body fat. It stores energy in the form of lipids (fats). It is also part of the endocrine system as it produces and stores hormones.

Adjuvant—often refers to a substance or treatment used in conjunction with the initial or primary cancer treatment.

Alpha-Hydroxyestrone—also called 16-Alpha-Hydroxyestrone. The hormone estrogen breaks down in the body into different forms called metabolites. Higher levels of 16-Alpha-Hydroxyestrone increase the risk of developing breast cancer, so it is sometimes called the "bad" estrogen. See Hydroxyestrone.

Angiogenesis—the process bodies use to grow blood vessels. Without a blood supply, cancers can't grow.

Anti-angiogenesis—interfering with the growth of new blood vessels, in particular those feeding tumors.

Anticancer—means "against cancer."

Anticarcinogen—refers to any chemical or compound that reduces the occurrence, severity, or risk of cancers.

Anti-inflammatory—has the ability to reduce inflammation.

Antimicrobial—kills or inhibits the growth of microorganisms such as bacteria, fungi, or protozoans.

Antimutagenic—has the ability to change genetic material.

Antioxidant—a substance that acts as a scavenger of free radicals, thus lessening or preventing oxidation (see Oxidation). Oxidative stress can lead to genetic damage that triggers cancer. See also Phenols and Flavonoids in the Nutrients section.

Antitumor—reduces the occurrence, severity, or risk of tumors.

Apoptosis—the programmed destruction of cells, which allows cancer cells to kill themselves without adversely affecting normal cells.

Biomarker—short for biological marker: something that can be measured to assess a biological state or health status.

Bisphenol A (BPA)—a manmade substance used to manufacture plastics. Linked to an increased risk of breast cancer and other cancers.

Carcinogenic—capable of causing cancer.

Cell adhesion—the binding of a cell to a surface. All organisms that are made up of more than one cell rely on correct cellular adhesion to create the structure of the organism.

Cell culture—process by which cells are grown under controlled conditions, generally in a laboratory. Often intended for scientific research.

Cell cycle—the process by which cells are created, grow, and die. In cancer, the cell cycle is abnormal. Cells divide to form new cells much more quickly than in normal tissue. The extra cells build up and form tumors.

Cell differentiation—process by which different cells in a multi-cellular organism (such as a human) take on different forms and functions.

Cell markers—biochemical or genetic attributes that are different for different types of cells.

Cell migration—movement of a group of cells from one place to another.

Cell proliferation—increase in the number of cells or growth in a certain cell type.

Chemopreventive—the use of chemical agents, drugs, or food nutrients to prevent the development of cancer.

Chemotherapy—the use of chemicals to target cancer cells.

Cohort study—an observational study that follows a population who do *not* have a particular disease, while comparing their life histories with people who have the disease. Usually performed to identify risk factors.

Correlational study—a type of observational study where the researchers look to see what factors in a person's life might be associated with certain outcomes, such as disease.

Cross-sectional study—a type of observational study where the researchers look at a population at one single moment in time to see what issues are most prevalent.

DNA—stands for deoxyribonucleic acid, a protein molecule that tells cells how to grow.

Dopamine—a hormone that acts as a neurotransmitter.

Ecological study—a type of observational study used to identify specific risk factors for a particular disease or other condition.

Endocrine—refers to both the endocrine organ system, which includes the ovaries in women and the testes in men and the thyroid, parathyroid, pituitary, adrenal, pineal, thymus, and hypothalamic glands in both sexes.

Estrogen-mediated cancer—a cancer that forms in tissue that has estrogen receptors, which are also called estrogen-sensitive, estrogen-dependent, hormone-related, or hormone-modified cancer.

Estrogen receptor—a protein molecule within a cell that will only bind to estrogen or an estrogen analog. Once estrogen binds to the receptor, it can signal changes in the cell.

Experimental study—a research study in which something is tested; for example, a trial of a drug or nutrient to see if it works against a particular disease.

Free radical—an atom, molecule, or ion that has a "dangling" (unattached) covalent bond. This makes it prone to binding to other atoms or molecules. When it binds to certain molecules within a cell, it can disrupt normal cell processes.

Genetically modified organism (GMO)—a life form that has had a change deliberately induced in its genetic makeup. See Mutation.

Herbicides—compounds that kill weeds and other unwanted plants. These chemicals are often toxic and many are classified as carcinogens.

Heterocyclic amine (HCA)—molecule containing a nitrogen group (amine) and at least two other elements. One type of HCA is a carcinogenic substance created by cooking meat at high temperatures.

High mammographic density—an area of dense breast tissue that shows up on a mammogram.

Hormones—chemical messengers made by the body and released into the blood where they are carried to other parts of the body.

Hydroxyestrone—also called 2-hydroxestrone. A metabolite of estrogen, often called the "good" estrogen. Higher levels of 2-hydroxyestrone are linked to a lower risk of developing breast cancer. See Alpha-Hydroxyestrone.

Hypomethylating—decreasing

Immune system—the body's defense system against disease.

In vitro study—an experimental study done on cells or molecules.

In vivo study—an experimental study done on living organisms, usually plants, animals, or humans.

Incidence—the rate at which something occurs: for example, the incidence of breast cancer in women over fifty.

Inflammation—the body's physical response to stress such as injury or infection, which can include pain, swelling, redness, and loss of function. While inflammation is a normal part of the immune system response to an acute injury or illness, chronic inflammation can cause permanent damage.

Insulin-like growth factor (IGF)—substance secreted by the liver that limits cell death (apoptosis). May play a role in stimulating breast cancer growth.

Intervention study—an experimental study in which a new treatment for a particular condition is tested. Usually done as a *randomized controlled* study, meaning that the subjects of the study are randomly divided into two groups. One group receives the intervention—the treatment being studied—and the other does not (they may get a *placebo* treatment that resembles the actual treatment, but is not expected to have any effect). The second group is the control group. The study tests whether or not the new treatment works better than the placebo.

Laboratory studies—any study done in a laboratory; usually refers to *in vitro* studies but some *in vivo* studies are also laboratory studies. Studies done in a laboratory usually can be strictly controlled so that unexpected variables do not affect the study.

Magnetic resonance imaging (MRI)—a type of scan that uses magnetism and radio waves instead of radiation to create a computerized image.

Malnutrition—physical state that results from not getting enough necessary nutrients. Not always the same thing as starvation, which is lack of sufficient calories to maintain life. People can be overweight and still malnourished if they are deficient in even one necessary nutrient.

Mammogram—image (-*gram*) taken of breast tissue (*mammo*- as in mammary) with an X-Ray, ultrasound, or MRI. Usually done to look for masses.

Menopause—the end of the fertile phase of a woman's life. Most women become capable of conceiving a child in the early teens and remain fertile for thirty to forty years. At the end of this time, the ovaries stop releasing eggs and the hormones that supported the uterus. Menses ("periods") stop and both the uterus and the ovaries begin to atrophy. Menopause can also be induced by surgical removal of the ovaries.

Meta-analysis—a review of several different studies on the same issue that evaluates differences and similarities in study results. An important tenet of the scientific method is that a study must be reproducible, which means a similar study should yield similar results. If it does not, there may have been problems with either study. The more studies that show similar results, the more likely it is that those results are meaningful.

Metabolism—the chemical reactions within the body that sustain life. Metabolism comprises two functions: catabolism (breakdown of components) and anabolism (creation of new components).

Metabolites—substances that result from catabolism of components. Estrogen metabolites, for example, result from the breakdown of the hormone estrogen.

Minimize—to reduce or possibly prevent.

Mutagenic—capable of causing changes in DNA that lead to mutations.

Mutation—a change in a gene that causes an organism to develop in a different way. Many mutations are spontaneous: they happen for reasons we don't understand. Mutation can also be induced, usually by chemicals or radiation. See GMO.

Neurotransmitter—Chemical made by the body that transmits signals throughout the nervous system effecting sleep, mood, and behavior. Over one hundred neurotransmitters have been identified.

Observational study—research that does not involve an experiment; the researchers do not test anything or try to change anything, they simply observe the study subjects and draw conclusions.

Oncogene—a mutated gene that has the potential to cause cancer.

Oncogenomics—the study of genes associated with cancer.

Oncology—medical specialty that studies and treats cancer. Cancer specialists are called oncologists.

Ontogenesis—the process by which a new organism comes into being and grows to maturity. Sometimes refers to the entire life span of an organism.

Organochlorides—a class of chemical compounds that contain chlorine. Many have been shown to have harmful effects on people or the environment.

Oxidation—a chemical reaction in cells that creates free radicals (see Free radical). Free radicals can trigger damaging changes in cells and even cause cell death. Cellular oxidation is a biological precursor to many cancers.

Oxidative stress—when the damage done by oxidation is greater than the body's ability to repair it.

Peer-reviewed—has been read and evaluated by experts in the same field.

Pesticides—compounds, generally chemically derived, that kill pests such as insects.

Plasma—usually, the yellow fluid component of blood that cells float in. Can also refer to the fluid in or around cells.

Polycyclic aromatic hydrocarbon (PAH)—a carcinogenic substance created when organic matter is not burned completely. Often found in cooked foods, especially meat.

Polymorphism—means "many forms." In biology, refers to two or more forms of any kind of organism that can result from a change in a gene.

Postmenopausal—after menopause is complete.

Premenopausal—the period leading up to menopause. Some women have noticeable emotional swings, changes in periods, and other physical changes for one or more years before menopause.

Recurrence—relapse, as when a cancer comes back after remission.

Replicative DNA polymerases—enzymes that enable DNA to reproduce.

Review study—see Meta-analysis.

Signal transduction—when certain molecules bind to a receptor site, either on the membrane of a cell or in the cell, they cause a signal to be sent to the cell. The signal may tell the cell to grow, divide, or even change its structure.

Signaling pathway—the chain of events that follows from a certain signal being given to a cell.

Significant association—a statistical term meaning that two or more things have been shown to be related in a way that is more than just chance. For instance, smoking tobacco has been shown to have a significant association with lung cancer.

Synergistic effect—when two or more things combine to have a greater effect than would be expected as a result of each separate thing.

Triple negative breast cancers—a group of cancers that are not hormone modified.

Tyrosine kinase receptors—cell receptors that play a critical role in the development of many cancers.

Nutrient Glossary

Nutrients play important roles in breast cancer prevention and treatment. They are cofactors in many biological processes throughout the body. Nutrient deficiencies not only cause malnutrition, but can hinder proper function of the endocrine and immune pathways and reduce the efficacy of medications.

Alpha-carotene—carotenes are nutrients made by plants; animals (including humans) do not make them and so have to eat the plants to get these nutrients. Alpha-carotene is a weak source of vitamin A. Higher blood levels of alpha-carotene are associated with a lower risk of death.

Anthocyanin—anthocyanins from peaches and plums reduce cell proliferation in estrogen-dependent breast cancer cells. See Flavonoid.

Beta-carotenes—red-orange, fat-soluble nutrients that are converted in the body to vitamin A.

Brassicas—genus of plants in the mustard family. Plants in this genus are also known as cruciferous vegetables, cabbages, or mustards.

Butyrates—compounds that provide food, energy, and protection for cells lining the colon.

Caffeic acid—a phenolic compound found in apples, arugula, and kale that shows promise in both preventing and inhibiting breast cancer growth.

Cannabidiol (CBD)—compound found in hemp. It does not have psychotropic compounds, tetrahydrocannabinol, or THC.

Carotenes—nutrients from plants that have antioxidant properties. See Carotenoids.

Carotenoids—broadly classified into two classes, *carotenes* (alpha-carotene, beta-carotene, and lycopene) and *xanthophylls* (beta-cryptoxanthin, lutein, and zeaxanthin). Alpha-carotene, beta-carotene, and beta-cryptoxanthin are provitamin A carotenoids, meaning they can be converted by the body to retinol, a form of vitamin A. Carotenoids also have antioxidant properties.

Catechins—nutrients found in tea, cocoa, and some fruits and vegetables. Catechins such as EGCG reduce the potential for environmental toxins to act as carcinogens in our bodies.

Docosahexaenoic acid (DHA)—a fatty acid primarily found in nuts, seeds and extracted from algae and sold in supplements that may also help increase the effect of chemotherapy on cancer cells.

Ellagic acid—a phenol found in fruits and vegetables that has antiproliferative and antioxidant properties.

Epigallocatechin-3-gallate (EGCG)—an antioxidant found in green tea that inhibits cancer development and reduces cell proliferation in existing tumors via an epigenetic effect.

Ferulic acid—a phenol found in coffee beans, apples, artichokes, peanuts, pineapple, oranges, rice, wheat, oats, and water chestnuts. It has antioxidant properties and may also have antitumor effects on breast cancer.

Fiber—the part of plant foods that acts as a prebiotic, feeding the probiotic organisms in our intestines. Both soluble and insoluble forms of fiber bind with toxins, increase cellular receptivity to insulin, and hold moisture in the intestines, which improves hydration.

Flavonoids—nutrients from plants that have antioxidant, antibacterial, and anti-inflammatory properties. *Isoflavonoids* are a form of flavonoid.

Flavonols—flavonoids that inhibit breast carcinogenesis. They are found in plant foods such as onion, kale, broccoli, lettuce, tomatoes, apples, grapes, berries, and tea. Include *isoflavones*.

Gingerol—active ingredient of ginger that breaks down into other compounds and is responsible for ginger's antinausea and antidiarrheal effects. Shogaol, one of the compounds formed from gingerol, also promotes apoptosis.

Glucosinolates—anticancer compounds found in concentration in cruciferous vegetables and pungent plants such as horseradish and mustard. Glucosinolates, a class of sulphur-containing glycosides, and their breakdown products, such as the isothiocyanates, are compounds involved in modulation of carcinogen-metabolizing enzyme systems.

Glycolipid—a combination of a lipid (fat) with a carbohydrate molecule. Used by the body for energy.

Hesperidin—flavonoid found in citrus fruits that may be particularly effective in preventing hormone-related cancers by interrupting hormone receptor binding in cancerous cells.

Indole-3-carbinol—nutrient found in brassica vegetables that may have anticarcinogenic effects.

Isothiocyanates—sulfur compounds found in cruciferous vegetables that provide effective breast cancer protection via detoxification, hormone binding, and antitumor properties.

Lignans and enterolignans—plant compounds associated with fiber that have antioxidant, anti-inflammatory, and anticancer properties. Lignans are especially important for those with hormone-sensitive breast cancer as they are structurally similar to estrogen and can bind to estrogen receptors, thus blocking the actions of estrogen in the body.

Limonene—a compound found in the peels of lemons and other citrus fruits that has epigenetic and anti-angiogenesis properties.

Lutein—a xanthophyll carotenoid found in green leafy vegetables, eggs, and animal fat that provides protection against benign breast disease (BBD), an independent risk factor for breast cancer, through anti-oxidative or antiproliferative mechanisms.

Lycopene—a carotenoid with the capacity to affect breast cancer as it inhibits cell proliferation, arrests the cell cycle in different phases, and increases apoptosis.

Melatonin—a hormone that helps regulate the sleep cycle; also has anti-inflammatory properties. Dysregulation of melatonin is believed to be a causative factor in breast cancer development for night workers, insomniacs, and those who suffer from chronic interrupted sleep.

Methoxycinnamic acid—see Ferulic acid.

Naringenin—a flavonoid found in citrus fruits and tomatoes that may have protective effects against damage from BPA and also promote apoptosis in cancer cells. It may be effective in the treatment of triple negative breast cancer.

Nobiletin—a flavonoid found in citrus fruits and in concentrated amounts in citrus fruit peels. The most studied properties of nobiletin are its anti-inflammatory, cholesterol-lowering, and anticancer activities. Nobiletin may have the potential to suppress metastasis of breast cancer.

Oligosaccharide—oligosaccharides are prebiotic carbohydrates that feed gut flora, supporting healthy growth of internal bacterial ecology.

Omega-3 fatty acids—polyunsaturated fatty acids found in whole foods such as flaxseed, chia seed, and avocados. These essential fats inhibit cell proliferation and induce of apoptosis in human breast cancer cells, especially the triple negative subtype.

Omega-6 fatty acids—polyunsaturated fatty acids found in corn, soybean, rapeseed, sunflower oils, and many other foods. A diet higher in omega-6 fatty acids and lower in omega-3 fatty acids may have negative health effects.

Phenols and polyphenols—phenols, polyphenols, and phenolics have antioxidant effects. Breast cancer survivors have a lower recurrence rate when their diets are rich in polyphenols from foods such as broccoli, turmeric, pomegranate, and green tea.

Phytic acid—a form of phosphorus found in some plants, especially seeds, cereals, and whole grains.

Phytochemical—a chemical made by a plant. Anticancer phytochemicals include cyanidin, delphinidin, quercetin, kaempferol, ellagic acid, resveratrol, and pterostilbene.

Phytoestrogens—plant compounds that are structurally similar to the human hormone estrogen which allows them to bind to sites on cells called estrogen receptors. They block estrogen from binding to the cells, which appears to reduce the chance of estrogen-stimulated cancer development.

Prebiotics—dietary fiber that may enhance growth of helpful bacteria in the lower digestive tract.

Probiotics—microorganisms from food or supplements that help restore a healthy balance of bacteria in the intestines.

Procyanidins—a type of flavonoid. Pentameric procyanidin, found in *Theobroma cacao*, inhibits growth of human breast cancer cells.

Quercetin—a phytoestrogen that can block estrogen from binding to estrogen receptor beta sites, protecting against the development of estrogen-stimulated cancer. Quercetin also helps mitigate the toxic effects of BPA, a known breast toxin.

Resveratrol—a nutrient that can block estrogen from binding to estrogen receptor beta sites, protecting against the development of metastatic breast cancer.

Sulforaphane—an isothiocyanate found in many brassica vegetables.

Tangeretin—flavone found in the peels of tangerines and other citrus fruits; known to trigger apoptosis in human breast cancer cells.

Vanillic acid—a derivative of ferulic acid found in honey, wine, and vinegar that inhibits human breast cancer cell growth.

Xanthophylls—carotenoid compounds that include beta-cryptoxanthin, lutein, and zeaxanthin.

RESOURCES

The following books and websites provide information about nutrition, toxins and/or microbes, and breast health.

BOOKS

Eat to Live: The Amazing Nutrient-Rich Program for Fast and Sustained Weight Loss, Revised Edition (Little, Brown and Company, 2011) By Joel Fuhrman

Healing Smoothies: 100 Research-Based, Delicious Recipes that Provide Nutrition Support for Cancer Prevention and Recovery (Skyhorse Press, 2015) By Daniella Chace

Plastic-Free: How I Kicked the Plastic Habit and How You Can Too (Skyhorse Press, 2012) By Beth Terry

The Cancer Recovery Plan: How to Increase the Effectiveness of Your Treatment and Live a Fuller, Healthier (Avery, 2005) By D. Barry Boyd and Marian Betancourt

The Cancer Survivor's Guide: Foods That Help You Fight Back (Book Publisher Company, 2009) By Dr. Neal Barnard and Jennifer K. Reilly

The China Study: The Most Comprehensive Study of Nutrition Ever Conducted And the Startling Implications for Diet, Weight Loss, And Long-term Health (BenBella Books, 2006) By Thomas Campbell and T. Colin Campbell

The Definitive Guide to Cancer, 3rd Edition: An Integrative Approach to Prevention, Treatment, and Healing (Celestial Arts, 2010) By Lise Alschuler, ND, FABNO, and Karloyn A. Gazella

The Definitive Guide to Thriving After Cancer - a Five Step Integrative Plan to Reduce the Risk of Recurrence and Build Lifelong Health (Ten Speed Press, 2013) By Lise Alschuler, ND, FABNO, and Karloyn A. Gazella

The Ecology of Breast Cancer: The Promise of Prevention and the Hope for Healing (CreateSpace, 2014) By Dr. Ted Schettler

What to Eat if You Have Cancer - Healing Foods that Boost Your Immune System (McGraw-Hill, 2006) By Maureen Keane and Daniella Chace

LABRATORY TESTING

Many clinics are just beginning to offer SNP, toxin and nutrient testing. At the time of publication of this book, many of the countries largest oncology clinics were starting to offer these tests that help guide personalized medicine. Because the list of clinics that provides these tests is changing rapidly, I will post up-to-date information on my website at daniellachace.com.

WEBSITES

The Washington Toxics Coalition (http://www.watoxics.org)
The Environmental Working Group (http://www. ewg.org)
Toxnet (http://www.toxnet.nlm.nih.gov)
ArtBeCause (http://www.artbecause.org)
The Human Food Project (http://www.humanfoodproject.com/ americangut/)

For more support in locating practitioners and clinics, laboratory tests, finding self-care resources, and keeping informed about integrative care, visit www. daniellachace.com

ABOUT THE AUTHOR

Daniella Chace, MS, CN, is a clinical nutritionist and educator. She is an expert in personalized medical nutrition therapy with an emphasis in toxicology, epigenetics, human microbial ecology, and orthomolecular applications in disease management.

She is the author of over twenty nutrition books, including *What to Eat if You Have Cancer* (McGraw-Hill, 2006), *More Smoothies for Life* (Clarkson Potter, 2007), and *Healing Smoothies for Cancer Recovery* (Skyhorse Press, 2015).

She is the creator of *NADb*, a medical nutrition research database. She is the host of NPR's *Nutrition Matters*. She lives in Port Townsend, Washington, where she sees clients in her private practice and develops recipes that support healing.

Learn more at www.daniellachace.com.

INDEX

A

ALAN. *See* Artificial light at night
    (ALAN)

Alcohol, 85, 87

Allium vegetables, 59, 66

Allspice, 79

Aluminum, 8, 21, 22, 23–24

Amalgam fillings, 28–29

Animal foods, 51, 86

Anthocyanins, 59–60, 69

Antibiotics, 51, 92–93, 96

Antimony, 21, 24–25

Antioxidants

    in apples, 67

    in apricots, 81

    in bananas, 67

    in beans, 68

    in berries, 59–60

    carotenoids as, 56

    in carrots, 69

    in chia seed, 75

    in citrus, 70

    in cocoa, 71

    in coconut oil, 76

    CoQ10 as, 101

    cysteine as, 104

    in guava, 72

    iodine as, 102–103

    licorice as, 103

    in mangoes, 73

    melatonin as, 112

    in melons, 74

    nutrients, 19

    in papaya, 77

    in peanuts, 77

    in potatoes, 78

    in rye, 84

    in spices, 79

    stress and, 115

    in tea, 61

    in tomatoes, 82

    in yeast, 74

Antiperspirants, 23–24

Apigenin, 73

Apoptosis, 57

Apples, 39, 67

Apricots, 61

Arsenic, 87

Arsenite, 21

Artificial light at night (ALAN), 104

Arugula, 60, 69

Ascorbic acid, 107

Aspartame, 88

Asthma medication, 19

Avocado oil, 76

Avocados, 67

B

Bacteria. *See* Microbes

Baked goods, 18

Bananas, 39, 67

Barium, 21

Basil, 32

Batteries, 25, 26

Beans, 68

Beets, 68

Bell peppers, 68

Berries, 59–60, 68–69

Betaine, 8

Bisphenol A (BPA), 36–40, 44, 106

Black cumin, 79

Black pepper, 79

Blood sugar, 48, 107

Blueberries, 6, 59

Bok choy, 60, 69

Borage, 75

BPA. *See* Bisphenol A (BPA)

Brassica vegetables, 60, 69

BRCA genes, 9, 25, 37

Bread, 18

Breast cancer subtypes, 4–7

Bromine, 17–19

Brussels sprouts, 60, 69

Burnt foods, 32

Butylparaben, 35

C

Cabbage, 60, 69

Cadmium, 21, 22, 25–26

Cake mix, 24

Caloric needs, 52

Caraway, 79

Carbohydrates, 47–49, 86–87

Cardamom, 79

Car interiors, 18

Carnosic acid, 5, 6, 73

Carotenoids, 55–57, 58

Carpet, 18

Carrots, 69–70

Catechins, 39

Catechol-O-methyltransferase (COMT), 10

Celery, 70

Cell division, 57

Chelation treatment, 22

Cherries, 39, 59

Chia seed, 75

Choline, 8

Chromium, 21

Cigarettes, 26, 32, 34

Cinnamon, 79

Citrus, 6, 39, 60, 70
Clostridium difficile, 96, 105
Cloves, 79
Cobalt, 21
Cocoa, 70–71
Coconut milk, 71
Coconut oil, 76–77
Coenzyme Q10 (CoQ10), 101
Coffee, 71, 85
Coffee creamer, 24
Collard greens, 60
Communication,
    non-violent, 115
COMT. *See* Catechol-O-
    methyltransferase (COMT)
Copper, 21
Corn, 83, 85
Creatine, 102
Cruciferous vegetables, 60
Cucumbers, 71
Cumin, 79
Curcumin, 5–6
Cysteine. *See* N-acetyl cysteine
    (NAC)

D
Dairy, 51, 85–86
Dental fillings, 28–29
Detoxification
    bisphenol A, 39
    defined, 15
    of PAHs, 33
    selenium in, 106–107
DetoxiGenomic Profile, 10, 30

DHA. *See* Docosahexanoic acid
    (DHA)
Diet. *See* Nutrition
Digestion
    internal ecology and, 96–97
    support, 45
Docosahexanoic acid (DHA), 7
Dopamine, 67
Dysbiosis, 93

E
EDCs. *See* Endocrine-disrupting
    chemicals (EDCs)
EGCG. *See* Epigallocatechin-3-
    gallate (EGCG)
Ellagic acid, 59
Endocrine-disrupting chemicals
    (EDCs), 4, 103
Environment,
    in epigenetics, 8
Epigallocatechin-3-gallate (EGCG),
    7, 82
Epigenetic microbes, 11–12
Epigenetics, 7–9
Ergosterol, 74
Erythritol, 81
EstroGenomic Profile, 13
Estrogen receptor negative breast
    cancer, 4, 5, 37, 43–44
Estrogen receptor positive breast
    cancer, 5, 95
Ethylparaben, 35
Excretion, of heavy metals, 31
Exercise, 111–112

F

Fabrics, 25

Fats, 52–55, 87–88

Fiber, dietary, 48, 68, 84

Figs, 61

Fillings, dental, 28–29

Fish, 28, 53

Flame retardants, 18, 25

Flavonols, 57–59, 68

Flaxseed, 75

Fluorescent bulbs, 28

Folate, 8, 39

Folic acid, 86

Food. *See* Nutrition

Food groups, 45–46

Fractionated pectin. *See* Modified citrus pectin (MCP)

Free radicals, 56. *See also* Antioxidants

Fruit. *See also specific fruits* citrus, 6, 39, 60, 70 stone, 61, 81

G

Garlic, 59, 66

Gene expression, 8–9

Genetics breast cancer subtypes and, 4–7 epigenetics in, 7–9 polymorphisms in, 9–11 toxins and, 8

Genetic tests, 3–4, 9–10

Ginger, 71

Glazes, 27

Glutamine, 10

Glutathione, 31

Glutathione S-transferases (GSTs), 10–11

Glycine, 10, 31

Grapefruit, 70

Greens, 72

Green tea, 7, 34, 61, 82

GSTs. *See* Glutathione S-transferases (GSTs)

Guava, 72

H

Hair products, 19

HCAs. *See* Heterocyclic amines (HCAs)

Heavy metals. *See also* Aluminum; Antimony; Cadmium; Lead; Mercury accumulation of, 21–22 breast cancer and, 20–21 as endocrine-disrupting chemicals, 4 in epigenetics, 8 examples of, 20 excretion of, 31 liver enzymes and, 10 reduction of, 30–32 sources of, 21 tests for, 29–30

Hemp seed, 75–76

HER2, 37

Herbs, 60, 73

Hesperidin, 70

Heterocyclic amines (HCAs), 33–34

HMP. *See* Human Microbiome Project (MHP)

Holy basil, 32

Hormones, endocrine-disrupting chemicals and, 4

Human Microbiome Project (MHP), 91, 100

Hydration, 82

Hyperglycemia, 48–49, 107

I

Inflammatory breast cancer (IBC), 23, 37

Insulin-like growth factor 1 (IGF-1), 80, 85, 88

Insulin resistance, 111–112

Iodine, 30–31

Iodine deficiency, 17–18, 102–103

Iodine supplementation, 102–103

ION (Individual Optimal Nutrition) Profile, 13

Isobutylparaben, 35

K

Kale, 60

Kefir, 39

Kimchi, 39

L

Lactobacillus, 94

Lactobacillus acidophilus, 94, 96, 105

Lactobacillus casei, 96

Lactobacillus plantarum, 97

Lactobacillus reuteri, 96–97

Lead, 8, 21, 26–27

Leeks, 59

Legumes, 51, 73

L-glutamic acid, 31

Licorice, 103

Light, artificial, 104

Lignans, 83

Liver enzymes, 10, 15

Lotion, 34

Lycopene, 70, 72, 82

M

Magnesium, 10

Maltitol, 81

Mangoes, 73

Massage, 113

Mattresses, 18

MCP. *See* Modified citrus pectin (MCP)

Meat, 33–34, 51, 86

Meditation, 113–114

Melatonin, 31, 39, 103–104, 112–113

Melons, 74

Mercury, 8, 21, 27–29

Metals. *See* Heavy metals

Metastasis, 102

Methionine, 8, 10

Methylation, 8, 11–12

Methyl group, 9

Methylobacterium radiotolerans, 94

Methylparaben, 35

Microbes
 antibiotics and, 92–93
 breast protective, 94
 digestion and, 92
 dysbiosis and, 93
 epigenetic, 11–12
 estrogens and, 92
 gut, 45
 infection and, 92
 initial colonization by, 92
 pathogenic, 94
 probiotics and, 94–96
Microbiome, 90–91
Microbiota, 90
Milk, 51, 85–86
Milk alternatives, 74
Mitochondrial function, 17
Modified citrus pectin (MCP), 102
Mouthwash, 19
Mustard greens, 60, 69
Mustard seed, 79

N

NAC. *See* N-acetyl cysteine (NAC)
N-acetyl cysteine (NAC), 10, 31,
 33, 104–105
Naringenin, 6
Nectarines, 61
Nickel, 21, 22
Night, artificial light in, 104
Non-violent communication
 (NVC), 115
Nutmeg, 80
Nutrition

breast cancer subtypes and, 5–7
carbohydrates in, 47–49
digestion support with, 45
epigenetics and, 8–9
estrogen receptor negative
 breast cancer and, 5
estrogen receptor positive
 breast cancer and, 5
fats in, 52–55
food groups in, 45–46, 46–47
goals of, 45
importance of, 43
mercury in, 28
microbes and, 95
plastic in, 38–39
protein in, 49–52
triple negative breast cancer
 and, 6–7
Nutritional yeast, 74
Nuts, 51, 74–75
NVC. *See* Non-violent
 communication (NVC)

O

Oats, 84
Obesity, 17, 35, 91, 114
Oils, 76–77
Oleanolic acid, 66, 73
Olive oil, 77
Omega-3 fatty acids, 6–7,
 53–55
Onions, 39, 59, 66
Organic label, 44
Overweight, 114

P

PAHs. *See* Polycyclic aromatic hydrocarbons (PAHs)

Paint, 26

Papaya, 77

Paprika, 80

Parabens, 4, 8, 34–35

Peaches, 61

Peanut oil, 77

Pectin. *See* Modified citrus pectin (MCP)

Pentameric procyanidin, 71

Personal care products, 34

Pesticides, 19, 44

PhIP, 33–34

Phthalates, 4, 8, 36–40. *See also* Bisphenol A (BPA)

Phthalates and Parabens Profile, 40

Pineapple, 77

Plant proteins, 49

Plastic, 26, 37, 38–39

Plumbing fixtures, 27

Plums, 61

Polycyclic aromatic hydrocarbons (PAHs), 10, 11, 32–33, 88

Polymorphisms, 9–11

Pomegranate, 77

Pool sanitizers, 19

Potassium bromate, 18

Potatoes, 77

Power food groups, 46–47

Prebiotics, 95

Primrose oil, 75

Probiotics, 94–96, 100, 105

Processed food, 44, 87

Propylparaben, 35

Protein, 49–52

Protein powder, 77

Prunes, 61

Pterostilbene, 6

Pumpkin seeds, 76

Q

Quercetin, 39, 59, 106

R

Radish, 60

Recurrence, carotenoids and, 55–56

Red meat, 51, 86

Resveratrol, 69

Riboflavin, 106

Rice, 84, 87

Rosemary, 5, 6, 32, 73, 80

Rye, 84

S

Saccharomyces boulardi, 105

Sacro-B, 105

Saffron, 80

Salt, 77

Seeds, 51, 74–76

Selenite, 21

Selenium, 27, 30–31, 106–107

Self-care

    exercise as, 111–112

    massage as, 113

    meditation as, 113–114

    optimal body-weight as, 114

Self-care (*Continued...*)
sleep as, 112–113
stress reduction as, 114–115
Sesame oil, 77
Sesame seeds, 76
Single nucleotide polymorphisms
(SNPs), 9–11
Sleep, 112–113
SNPs. *See* Single nucleotide
polymorphisms (SNPs)
Soap, 34
Soft drinks, 19
Solid fats, 87–88
Sphingomonas yanoikuyae, 94
Spices, 60, 79–80
Spinach, 72
Squash, 80–81
Stone fruit, 61, 81
Stool test, 100
Strawberries, 59
Stress reduction, 114–115
Subtypes, of breast cancer, 4–7
Sucralose, 88
Sugar, 48–49, 93
Sulfur nutrients, 31
Sunflower seeds, 76
Sunscreen, 24
Supplements
CoQ10, 101
creatine, 102
iodine, 102–103
licorice, 103
melatonin, 103–104
modified citrus protein, 102

N-acetyl cysteine, 104–105
for phthalate toxicity, 40
probiotic, 105
quercetin, 106
riboflavin, 106
selenium, 106–107
vitamin C, 107
vitamin D3, 107–108
zinc, 108–109
Sweeteners, 81, 88
Sweet potatoes, 78
Synthetic sweeteners, 88

T
Tamoxifen, 101, 106, 113
Tea, 7, 34, 39, 61, 82
Tests
genetic, 3–4, 9–10
for heavy metals, 29–30
for toxins, 16–17
Thermometers, 28
Thyme, 73
Tin, 21
TNBC. *See* Triple negative breast
cancer (TNBC)
Tomatoes, 82
Toothpaste, 19, 24
Toxic Element Clearance Profile,
29–30
Toxins. *See also* Detoxification
defined, 15
elimination of, 15
epigenetic, 8
laboratory tests for, 16–17

Trans fats, 52, 87

Triple negative breast cancer
(TNBC), 6–7, 53–55, 112

Turmeric, 5, 32, 80

V

Vanadate, 21

Vanilla beans, 80

Vegetable oil, 19

Vegetables. *See also specific vegetables*
allium, 59, 66
brassica, 60, 69

Vegetables, carotenoids in,
55–56

Vitamin A, 56

Vitamin B2, 106

Vitamin B6, 11

Vitamin B12, 8

Vitamin C, 107

Vitamin D3, 107–108

Vitamin D deficiency, 107

W

Walnut oil, 77

Walnuts, 76

Water, 82

Weight, 114

Whole grains, 83–84

X

Xenoestrogens, 33

Xylitol, 81

Y

Yeast, nutritional, 74

Z

Zinc, 30–31, 76, 108–109

ALSO AVAILABLE

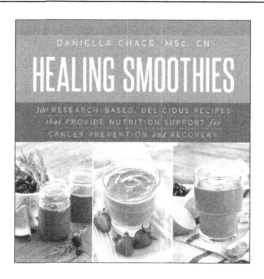

Healing Smoothies

100 Research-Based, Delicious Recipes That Provide Nutrition Support for Cancer Prevention and Recovery

Daniella Chace, MSc, CN

Fight cancer and help prevent recurrence with these delicious smoothies!

There has been a tremendous surge in research identifying the specific nutrients that have the ability to change the course of cancer. With a clearer understanding of the role that food nutrients, toxins, and microflora play in disease prevention and development, we have some of the long sought answers to our questions about what triggers, promotes, heals, and prevents cancer. Chace offers medicinally-potent smoothie recipes that taste great and provide cancer protective and healing nutrients, such as:

- Banana Coconut Cocoa Cream

- Banana Ginger Dream

- Basil Berry Citrus

- Tangerine Currant Citrus

- Watermelon Blackberry and Ginger

The ingredients section of the book provides more than sixty cancer-healing foods that are perfect smoothie additions. Cancer patients and their care providers can use these smoothie recipes or create their own from the ingredients list to help heal and nourish the patient throughout the treatment process. In addition, many of the nutrients in these smoothies have been found to support remission and reduce the risk for cancer recurrence.

$16.99 Hardcover • ISBN 978-1-63220-447-9

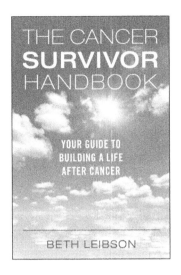

The Cancer Survivor Handbook

Your Guide to Building a Life After Cancer

Beth Leibson

You've beat cancer, and now it's time to face the rest of your life—here are all your questions, answered.

The Cancer Survivor Handbook is a companion and guide for those millions of individuals who are finally done with treatments but are still on the journey to wholeness. Beth Leibson completed her chemotherapy and radiation in 2007. She had beat cancer, but was left with lingering memory issues, exhaustion, depression, pain, and the fear that at any point, the cancer could return. Here she tells the story of how she rebuilt her life, and shares advice from other experts, addressing the emotional, medical, and professional challenges of life after cancer. Here are the questions you're afraid to ask ("When will my sex drive come back?"), the questions you hadn't yet considered ("How do I reenter the work force after a 'break' of a year or more?"), and those you know you should be thinking about but haven't had the energy for ("What supplements or alternative therapies should I be taking to regain my strength?").

Warm, honest, and full of sage advice, this is the book Leibson wishes she had had when the nightmare of cancer treatments drew to a close and the overwhelming reality of starting life over again began.

$17.95 Paperback • ISBN 978-1-62873-613-7

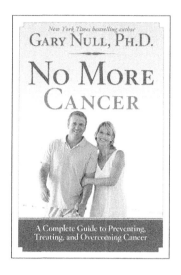

No More Cancer

A Complete Guide to Preventing, Treating, and Overcoming Cancer

Gary Null, PhD

Fight cancer the natural way!

One word strikes more fear into a person's mind than any other: CANCER. The physical, mental, emotional, and financial toll that comes with a cancer diagnosis is immense and affects not only cancer patients but also families and entire communities. The vast majority of individuals who lose the battle against cancer are treated with the standard orthodox therapy. These people may never have questioned their oncologists, believing that they were in the best possible hands with their physicians' advanced education, knowledge of latest treatments, and all the tools of modern research at their disposal.

In this groundbreaking book, Gary Null debunks the commonly accepted belief that drugs and chemotherapy are the only cures for cancer and explores the alternative treatments that most mainstream doctors will never discuss with their patients. Dr. Null asserts that there are foods and supplements that boost the body's immune system and can actually prevent and reverse cancer. Did you know that eating lemons and melons can help balance your body's pH, which will help prevent and treat cancer? You knew that fiber is important for a healthy diet, but did you know that it lowers the risk of breast, colorectal, uterine, and prostate cancers? Have you heard of maitake mushrooms, which kill cancer cells by enhancing the activity of T-helper cells? In addition to diet, Dr. Null discusses important supplements and herbs and cutting-edge therapies you may never have heard of. With twenty-five cancer-fighting recipes and testimonials from individuals who have found health through Dr. Null's methods, this book could save your life.

$24.95 Hardcover • ISBN 978-1-62087-617-6